# Innovations in Nursing Education:
## Building the Future of Nursing
### VOLUME 3

*Edited by:*
**Linda Caputi,** EdD, RN, CNE, ANEF

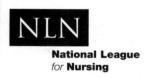

**National League**
*for* **Nursing**

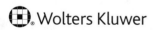

Philadelphia · Baltimore · New York · London
Buenos Aires · Hong Kong · Sydney · Tokyo

*Acquisitions Editor:* Sherry Dickinson
*Product Development Editor:* Meredith L. Brittain
*Editorial Assistant:* Dan Reilly
*Production Project Manager:* Marian Bellus
*Design Coordinator:* Joan Wendt
*Illustration Coordinator:* Jennifer Clements
*Manufacturing Coordinator:* Karin Duffield
*Marketing Manager:* Carolyn Fox

Copyright © 2016 National League for Nursing

9 8 7 6 5 4 3 2 1

Printed in the United States of America

**Library of Congress Cataloging-in-Publication Data**

Innovations in nursing education : building the future of nursing /
Linda Caputi, editor ; illustrations by Jennifer Clements.
    p. ; cm.
Includes bibliographical references.
ISBN 978-1-934758-22-9 (alk. paper)
    I. Caputi, Linda, editor of compilation.   II. National League for Nursing, issuing body.
    [DNLM: 1. Education, Nursing–organization & administration.
2. Education, Nursing–trends. WY 18]
    RT76
    610.73071′1–dc23               2013031359

DRC0915

# About the Editor

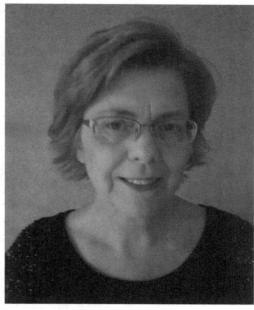

**Dr. Caputi** is the editor of the *Innovation* Center, a column in the National League for Nursing (NLN) journal *Nursing Education Perspectives*. She is a certified nurse educator and a fellow in the NLN's Academy of Nursing Education. Dr. Caputi is Professor Emeritus, College of DuPage, and she most recently taught an online master's in nursing education program. She has won six awards for teaching excellence from Sigma Theta Tau and is included in three different years in *Who's Who Among America's Teachers*. The second edition of her book *Teaching Nursing: The Art and Science* was selected as the winner of the 2010 Top Teaching Tools Award in the print category from the *Journal of Nursing Education*. She has served on the NLN's Board of Governors. Dr. Caputi is the president of Linda Caputi, Inc., a nursing education consulting company, and has worked with hundreds of nursing programs over the past 20 years on topics related to revising curriculum, transforming clinical education, test item writing, and test construction, using an evidence-based model for NCLEX® success, assisting with accreditation, and numerous other nursing education topics. She has recently co-authored the book *Mastering Concept-Based Teaching: A Guide for Nurse Educators* with Drs. Jean Giddens and Beth Rodgers, which is published by Elsevier. Dr. Caputi also is the editor of other books published through the NLN and Wolters Kluwer, including the first and second volumes of *Innovations in Nursing Education: Building the Future of Nursing* published in 2014 and 2015 and the *Certified Nurse Educator Review Book: The Official NLN Guide to the CNE Exam* published in 2015.

# About the Contributors

**Norah M. M. Airth-Kindree, DNP, MSN, RN,** is an assistant professor of nursing at the University of Wisconsin—Eau Claire. Norah practiced professional nursing in a variety of settings prior to embarking on an academic role in 2004, teaching primarily in the BSN completion program. Norah's area of scholarship and passion within nursing is public health. She was the recipient of the Mary Adelaide Nutting Award from the Wisconsin Public Health Association in 2013 for enhancing linkages between education and practice in the public health setting.

**Lori Arietta, MSN/Ed, RN,** has taught clinical education at Cleveland State University and at the community college level. Lori also worked full-time in a new BSN program, where her efforts focused on the development and implementation of the clinical coordinator position. During this time, she assisted the dean of the School of Nursing on several projects, including accreditation of the program. In addition to her clinical teaching experience, Lori practiced as an enterostomal therapy nurse and was recognized for her work with colorectal patients. She was the recipient of the Best of the Best in Nursing, 2008.

**Alyce S. Ashcraft, PhD, RN, CNE, ANEF,** is a tenured professor, recipient of the Roberts Endowed Practiceship in Nursing, and associate dean for research at the Texas Tech University Health Sciences Center in Lubbock, Texas. Her program of research focuses on preventing transfer of geriatric residents from skilled nursing to acute care, as well as implementation of evidence-based practice protocols in the clinical setting. After practicing in acute care, Alyce became a nurse educator, teaching ADN, BSN, MSN, and DNP students in traditional and nontraditional settings.

**Deborah R. Bambini, PhD, WHNP-BC, CNE, CHSE, ANEF,** is an associate professor at Grand Valley State University, where she has taught for more than 20 years. Her scholarly interests are focused on nursing education and strategies to enhance teaching effectiveness, which has led to a research program directed at best practices for simulation in nursing education. She also chaired the task force for curriculum revision, which resulted in a concept-based curriculum with simulation integrated throughout the undergraduate program. Deborah is a health information technology scholar, a simulation educator leader, and a fellow in the NLN Academy for Nursing Educators. She has presented her work at several national and international nursing education, interprofessional education, and simulation conferences and has published in various professional peer-reviewed journals and texts.

**Regina Bentley, EdD, RN, CNE,** has 25 years of teaching experience in health professions education, as well as 10 years of curriculum development and evaluation. She currently serves as an assistant dean for academic affairs and accreditation in the Texas A&M Health Science Center College of Medicine, as well as the director for the Education for Healthcare Professionals master's degree. She is responsible for monitoring curriculum development and coordinating the assessment of student learning outcomes. Regina's research is focused on interprofessional education, particularly assessing medical students' collaboration and teamwork.

**Carol Boswell, EdD, RN, CNE, ANEF,** is a tenured professor and recipient of the James A. "Buddy" Davidson Charitable Foundation Endowed Chair for Evidence-Based Practice at Texas Tech University Health Sciences Center School of Nursing. She has authored multiple publications related to evidence-based practice, mentoring, online teaching, and research. She has two published textbooks related to evidence-based practice in the areas of research and teaching. Carol has been an educator for more than 20 years, working at multiple levels, including ADN, RN-BSN, graduate, and continuing education. Carol was inducted as a fellow in the inaugural cohort for the NLN Academy of Nursing Education. She holds a certification as a nurse educator through the NLN. Carol is a strong advocate for effective faculty and peer mentoring.

**Steve Branham, PhD, RN, ACNP-BC, FNP-BC, FAANP,** has more than 32 years of progressive healthcare delivery experience and is a fellow in the American Association of Nurse Practitioners. Steve's contributions have included professor, manager, business owner, and CEO. He completed doctoral work at Texas Woman's University in 2011. Steve is an assistant professor in the Acute Care Nurse Practitioner program at Texas Tech University and serves as adjunct faculty at Texas Woman's University. Steve maintains an active clinical practice focused on critical and emergency care.

**Kellie Bruce, PhD, RN, FNP-BC,** is an assistant professor at Texas Tech University Health Sciences Center School of Nursing. She is the program director for the Family Nurse Practitioner track. She has been an RN for 27 years and an FNP for 15 years. Her areas of practice include adult cardiology and chronic illness treatment. Her areas of scholarship primarily relate to adult health and the use of simulation in APRN distance education programs.

**Margaret J. Bull, PhD, RN,** is a professor at Marquette University in Milwaukee, Wisconsin. She has more than 25 years of teaching experience and teaches research to undergraduate and graduate students in nursing. With the increased focus on evidence-based practice, she is committed to facilitating undergraduate students in appraising evidence for its relevance to clinical practice.

**Mary Ann Cantrell, PhD, RN, CNE,** is a professor in the College of Nursing at Villanova University. Mary Ann has been a faculty member at Villanova University for the past 25 years. Her program of clinical research addresses health-related quality-of-life outcomes for childhood cancer survivors. She has been involved in simulation-based research since 2005. Mary Ann's area of simulation-based research is focused on safety practices and clinical judgment skills in undergraduate students. In addition, she is a co-investigator in a Robert Wood Johnson–sponsored research investigation examining the research and scholarship productivity of doctorally prepared nursing faculty and the conflicting demands on them to teach and mentor doctoral students while establishing and maintaining their programs of research and scholarship.

**Terri A. Cavaliere, DNP, RN, NNP-BC,** is an assistant clinical professor in the School of Nursing at Stony Brook University in New York. She also maintains a clinical practice as an NP in a level-three neonatal intensive care unit. In addition to more than 20 years of teaching in a university setting and 30 years as an NNP, Terri is a nationally recognized author, consultant, and speaker. Her research areas include ethics and moral distress. She was instrumental in introducing team-based learning into an asynchronous distance graduate program in nursing. She has served as a member of the Council on Ethical Practice in Nursing for the New York State Nurses' Association; as president of the Long Island Association of Neonatal Nurses; as a member of the Board of Directors and NNP certification examination content team of the National Certification Corporation for Obstetric, Gynecologic, and Neonatal Nurses; and as a member of the Executive Council of the National Association of Neonatal Nurse Practitioners. In 2014, she received a Lifetime Achievement Award from the National Association of Neonatal Nurses.

**Virginia A. Coletti, PhD, RN, NPP, CS, CARN,** is a clinical associate professor in the School of Nursing at Stony Brook University in New York. She is a psychiatric NP/clinical nurse specialist in psychiatric mental health and a certified addictions RN. She has served on the Addictions Nursing Certification Board since 2008 and is a long-standing active member of Sigma Theta Tau in the Kappa Gamma Chapter. Virginia received her MSN from Stony Brook University and her PhD in education from La Salle University in Louisiana. Her doctoral study investigation was focused on the attitudes of nursing students toward people who are homeless. Her clinical program of scholarship is focused on addressing the needs of individuals experiencing stress related to diabetes, bereavement, and homelessness. She teaches in both the undergraduate and graduate Psychiatric Mental Health and the Master's in Education nursing programs.

**Vaneta M. Condon, PhD, MSN, RN,** is an associate professor emeritus at Loma Linda University School of Nursing in Loma Linda, California. She was an instructor in medical-surgical nursing and director of the skills lab for many years. She was instrumental in the development of the Learning Assistance Program, where she was the director until 2008. The development and implementation of The Exam Analysis© was a significant focus of her nursing career since 1983. Vaneta was the director of one state and two federal grants. These grants focused on assisting students from disadvantaged backgrounds to complete their nursing education and become licensed RNs. In addition, she and her husband served as medical missionaries in the Philippines for 7 years.

**Sarah W. Craig, PhD, MSN, RN, CCNS, CCRN, CSC,** is a certified clinical nurse specialist and assistant professor at the University of Virginia School of Nursing. She is a 2014 PhD graduate from the University of Virginia School of Nursing, a 2006 BSN graduate from Virginia Commonwealth University, and a 2005 diploma graduate from Danville Regional Medical Center School of Nursing. Sarah's teaching experience includes clinical instruction in acute care for undergraduate nursing students and graduate clinical nurse specialist students, APRN roles 1 and 2 for graduate nursing students, and a health assessment laboratory for undergraduate nursing students. Sarah is interested in professional development, as well as acute and critical care with a strong emphasis on cardiology and respiratory systems. She aspires to contribute to the learning needs of our students at the university to prepare them for the complex and wonderful world of nursing.

**Kathleen DeLeskey, DNP, RN, CNE, FJBI,** is an associate professor of nursing at Lawrence Memorial/Regis College in Medford, Massachusetts. In addition, she is a course coordinator for Fundamentals of Nursing for the evening division. Kathleen has more than 30 years of nursing experience, overwhelmingly as a perianesthesia nurse, and currently serves as the president of the Massachusetts Society of PeriAnesthesia Nurses. She is also co-chair of the Nursing Research Council at Hallmark Health in Medford, Massachusetts.

**Carol B. Della Ratta, PhD, CCRN,** is a full-time clinical assistant professor in the School of Nursing at Stony Brook University in New York. She has 25 years of experience teaching in undergraduate basic, accelerated, and RN-to-BSN programs. Carol's most recent efforts focus on active learning strategies such as on-site and distance team-based learning and simulation experiences. She has participated in the design and piloting of an interprofessional simulation experience for senior nursing and medical students at Stony Brook University. Her research interest includes new graduate nurses' experiences caring for patients with deteriorating statuses. Carol also serves as a nurse resident facilitator at the Stony Brook Medicine, UHC/AACN Nurse Residency Program.

**Emily Drake PhD, RN, FAAN,** is an associate professor at the University of Virginia School of Nursing, where she has served in leadership positions as an interim assistant dean, chair of the faculty organization, and director of the BSN program. The focus of her teaching, practice, and research is on maternal-child health and technology. She has more than 25 years of experience that includes practice as a staff nurse, a clinical specialist, and educator.

**Diane M. Ellis, MSN, RN, CCRN,** has been a clinical assistant professor at Pennsylvania's Villanova University College of Nursing for the past 10 years, working primarily with second degree students in accelerated programs with both teaching and administrative responsibilities. Her classroom and clinical teaching areas of focus are neuroscience and leadership nursing. She was a member of the Edmond J. Safra Visiting Nurse Faculty Program in Parkinson's Disease first cohort in 2009. Prior to joining Villanova University College of Nursing, Diane worked with Studer Group, a private healthcare consulting company, where she coached senior management and frontline staff in service excellence. Diane has extensive experience practicing as a neurological clinical nurse specialist.

**Kathleen M. Gambino, EdD, RN,** is a clinical associate professor in the School of Nursing at Stony Brook University in New York. As the program director for the RN-to-BSN program, she is involved in the development of curriculum and clinical opportunities aimed at meeting the unique needs of the associate to BSN student. Kathleen assisted in the establishment of a team-based learning platform for on-site and distance-learning nursing education. She is involved in designing an interprofessional simulation experience for RN and medical students. Kathleen is a member of the Stony Brook University's Institutional Review Board. Her research interests also include incivility in nursing education and the transition and retention of new graduate nurses to professional practice.

**Joanna Guenther, PhD, RN, FNP-BC, CNE,** is an associate professor of clinical nursing in the graduate program at the University of Texas School of Nursing in Austin. In addition to 15 years of online and classroom teaching experience, she holds certification as an FNP since 1996. By being committed to both education and practice, she maintains a special interest in integrating the classroom and clinical settings for future NPs. She utilizes and teaches evidence-based quality improvement and healthcare transformation by promoting care that is effective, safe, and efficient.

**Victoria R. Hammer, EdD, MN, RN, CNE,** is an associate professor of nursing at St. Cloud State University in Minnesota. She teaches the second-semester junior course Nursing Care of the Older Adult, oncology and end-of-life concerns in a senior medical-surgical course, and in a senior leadership/capstone seminar and clinical. She has taught in both ADN and BSN programs. Her longitudinal research study examines students' perceptions of cultural and interprofessional implications for nursing care in end-of-life simulations, as well as the impact of the simulations on the nursing care provided by students during the nursing program and as new graduate nurses. Victoria received her BSN from St. Olaf College in Northfield, Minnesota; her MSN from the University of Washington in Seattle; and her doctorate in education from the University of South Dakota in Vermillion. She is a member of Sigma Theta Tau International Honor Society of Nursing.

**Carmen V. Harrison, MSN, RNC,** is a PhD student at the University of Missouri—Kansas City. In addition, she is an associate professor at Good Samaritan College of Nursing and Health Science in Cincinnati, Ohio. Carmen has taught at the college for 12 years, where she has been committed to improving student learning outcomes through the use of active teaching-learning strategies. She has presented at regional and national nursing education conferences, disseminating her knowledge regarding innovative teaching methods and diversity within nursing education. Carmen's research interest is the critical thinking development of undergraduate nursing students in a concept-based nursing curriculum. Carmen also practices as a women's healthcare NP.

**Desiree Hensel, PhD, RN, PCNS-BC, CNE,** is an associate professor at the Indiana University School of Nursing. Her distinct body of research explores the use of innovative teaching strategies to help students acquire the profession's knowledge, skills, and attitudes in both clinical and classroom settings while more closely examining how nurses define themselves in the 21st century. Dr. Hensel has expertise with mixed-method approaches to evaluate learning outcomes and explore phenomena of interest to the profession of nursing. She has published extensively in top-tier nursing journals and has disseminated her work in national forums. She also co-edits the student-centered testing resource, Lippincott's NCLEX-RN Q&A.

**Susan M. Herm, MSN, RN-BC,** is an associate professor of nursing at St. Cloud State University in Minnesota. She teaches junior medical-surgical nursing courses and has taught at all levels of the BSN program at St. Cloud. She has taught in both ADN and BSN programs for more than 20 years and has worked in a variety of medical and surgical settings in both urban and rural areas. She recently completed a sabbatical project focusing on using simulation in nursing education. Susan is nationally certified through the American Association of Colleges of Nursing in medical-surgical nursing. She received her BSN from Winona State University and her MSN from the University of Minnesota. She is a member of Sigma Theta Tau International Honor Society of Nursing and the National League of Nursing.

**Meredith Hertel, BA, MAE,** is an instructor and undergraduate advisor in the Department of Art Education at Virginia Commonwealth University (VCU). In addition to teaching and mentoring undergraduate students, Meredith has directed a community contemporary art program called *Investigation NOW* for Richmond adolescents since 2013. Her research interests include how art can be used as a tool to spur cross-disciplinary dialogue and how contemporary art specifically fosters intellectual risk-taking behaviors in students. Meredith has participated in the Art of Nursing research initiative during her graduate studies at VCU since 2011.

**Peggy Hewitt, MSN, RN,** is a clinical assistant professor at the University of North Carolina at Greensboro (UNC-G) and a DNP student at Case Western Reserve University in Cleveland, Ohio. Her nursing career began as an ADN. She continued through an RN-BSN program and then proceeded to obtain an MSN. She teaches in the undergraduate program at UNC-G, in both the pre-licensure and RN-BSN programs. Peggy has 6 years of teaching experience and a passion for RN-BSN students and clinical education.

**Caralise W. Hunt, PhD, RN,** is an assistant professor in the Auburn University School of Nursing in Alabama. She teaches medical-surgical nursing in the undergraduate program. Her research interest is self-management behaviors of people living with type 2 diabetes mellitus. Caralise is chair of the Undergraduate Curriculum Committee for the School of Nursing and has an interest in curriculum development and curricular issues.

**Dana Hunt, DNP, MPH, RN,** is an associate professor in the graduate program at Southwest Baptist University, Mercy College of Nursing and Health Sciences. Dana has been a nurse for 19 years, earning degrees in both nursing and public health. Her experience is varied in nursing education and online learning, educational leadership, public health project coordination, diabetes education, critical care, and emergency nursing. Dana's research interests include public health, health promotion, nursing education, and online learning. As an NLN LEAD program alumni, Dana is committed to teaching graduate nursing students to embrace lifelong learning, leadership development, and the knowledge to transform our healthcare system utilizing evidence-based practice.

**Brenda L. Janotha, DNP-DCC, ANP-BC, APRN,** is an assistant professor at Columbia University School of Nursing in New York City and teaches in the graduate nursing practice program. In addition to teaching, she has maintained a clinical practice as an adult NP in primary care for more than 16 years. Brenda is a candidate for her second doctorate, an EdD in human development and educational psychology, at Hofstra University. She is committed to improving teaching and learning strategies and has a research track in evaluating student outcomes. She presents regionally and nationally on her educational research.

**Lee-Ellen C. Kirkhorn, PhD, RN,** is a professor and chair of nursing at Indiana University—Purdue University in Fort Wayne, Indiana. Her present emphasis is teaching Evidence-Based Practice and Research in Healthcare at the baccalaureate level and Legal and Ethical Considerations at the doctoral (DNP) level. She also serves as an advisor and mentor to master's students. Lee-Ellen possesses more than three decades of experience as a nurse educator and 19 years of experience as an adult-gerontology primary care NP. Her area of research includes ethical practices among practicing RNs.

**Katherine A. Koepke, MS, BSN, RN, CNHP,** currently serves as the nursing science lab coordinator at St. Cloud State University in Minnesota. She assists with training and simulation learning in a variety of baccalaureate nursing courses. In addition, Katherine is responsible for the budget for the nursing skills lab and the running of the day-to-day operations in the nursing lab. She has been an RN and educator for many years in a variety of medical and educational settings. She is certified in natural health and parish nursing, as well as an Epic Inpatient Trainer. Kathy received her BSN from the College of St. Scholastica in Duluth, Minnesota. She obtained her master's degree in human resources, staff development, and training from St. Cloud State University. She has done missionary work in Honduras and has been a keynote speaker at several conferences. Katherine is a member of Sigma Theta Tau International Honor Society of Nursing.

**Karen A. Landry, PhD, RN,** received her doctorate in nursing science from Texas Woman's University and her MSN and BSN from Northwestern State University in Shreveport, Louisiana. She has an active nursing license in the state of Texas, as well as inactive licenses in Louisiana and Arkansas. Karen has taught undergraduate and graduate nursing courses for 20 years and has more than 30 years of clinical practice. Her work focuses in the area of ethics, nursing education, quality of life, and interprofessional healthcare education and simulation. She has published in the *Annals of Behavioral Science and Medical Education, Nurse Educator, Innovations in Nursing Education,* and at the university level. Karen has presented at Sigma Theta Tau International, American Association of Heart Failure Nurses, National Nursing Ethics, HIMSS Nursing Informatics Symposium, Annals of Behavioral Science and Medical Education, Southern Group on Educational Affairs, American Academy on Communication in Healthcare, and AACN Baccalaureate Education conferences.

**Kezia D. Lilly, DNP, MBA HC, RN,** is an associate professor in nursing and dean at Mercy College of Nursing and Health Sciences of Southwest Baptist University in Springfield, Missouri. She has worked in higher education for nearly 5 years, with the past 3 years spent in higher education administration. For the past 15 years, Kezia has worked in a full array of managed care positions, including pre-certification, case management, disease management, physician and facility auditing, quality improvement, data analysis, quality reporting and clinical-driven administrative presentations, project management, quality reviews, and appeals. She has worked in data analytics for more than 10 years. As a consultant and nurse, Kezia has worked on several medical management, clinical database, and analysis projects, including collaboration with hospital systems, ambulatory care centers, and integrated health systems across the country. She has an extensive background in providing project management for new system implementations and has developed integrated links with the electronic health record (EHR) systems of major providers. Additionally, she has consulted nationally with EHR organizations to provide input on development from the nurse user perspective. In nursing and healthcare education, Kezia is dedicated to building positive leaders now and in the future.

**Susan L. Lindner, MSN, RNC-OB,** is an assistant clinical professor in the School of Nursing at Virginia Commonwealth University (VCU). In addition to teaching undergraduate nursing students didactic and clinical, she is the founder of the VCU School of Nursing Doula Program, offering doula services to the underserved population in Richmond. Susan introduced a pilot art visualization learning activity to students that laid the foundation for the Art of Nursing research initiative. She has 10 years of experience teaching undergraduate baccalaureate nursing students with an emphasis in women's health, health assessment, and community health.

**Carley G. Lovell, MA, MS, RN, WHNP-BC,** is a PhD student at Medical University of South Carolina and a clinical assistant professor at Virginia Commonwealth University School of Nursing in Richmond, Virginia. She teaches in the undergraduate nursing program in the clinical areas of Technologies of Nursing, Nursing of Women, and Health Assessment. Carley provides clinical oversight of student and faculty dyads participating in the Art of Nursing research initiative. Her research interests include biobehavioral symptom science in the area of obesity and binge eating/drinking, with the goal of advancing etiological understanding of the behavior and identifying personalized strategies to reduce maladaptive coping binge responses. Carley practices as a women's health NP at a weight loss and wellness clinic as well.

**Claire Malinowski, BSN, RN,** is a pediatric trauma nurse. Following graduation from Indiana University School of Nursing, she spent 3 years working in the emergency department and pediatric intensive care unit at Vanderbilt Children's Hospital. She currently works in the emergency department at Cincinnati Children's Hospital Medical Center.

**Iris Mamier, PhD, MSN, RN,** is an assistant professor in the graduate program at Loma Linda University School of Nursing in California. She teaches research courses in the master's and DNP programs, as well as Philosophy of Nursing Science in the PhD program. Iris has taught and directed the Pipeline Program at Loma Linda University School of Nursing for 3 years. This program seeks to provide educational access to baccalaureate nursing students from minority or disadvantaged backgrounds and to facilitate their academic success. For several years, Iris has been involved with the Learning Assistance Program, where she successfully worked with students who wanted to improve the effectiveness of their studying and exam-taking skills using The Exam Analysis©, a tool described in this book. She also helped to develop a course and mentored students after an academic failure experience. Nursing student retention issues continue to hold her research interest as she mentors doctoral students while also engaging in scholarship in the area of spirituality and health care, with specific interest in nursing spiritual care.

**Bette Mariani, PhD, RN,** is an assistant professor in the College of Nursing at Villanova University. Bette's research agenda includes simulation-based research, which is focused on safety practices, medication administration, clinical judgment skills in undergraduate students, outcomes of debriefing, simulation instrument development and psychometric testing, and standardized patients with disabilities. Bette is a member of the INACSL Research Committee, the subcommittee chair of the INACSL Research Monitoring Subcommittee, and a member of the INACSL Standards Committee on Simulation Design.

**Yondell Masten, PhD, WHNP-BC, RNC-OB,** is a tenured professor, recipient of the Hall Endowed Chair for Nursing Excellence in Women's Health, and the associate dean for outcomes management and evaluation at the Texas Tech University Health Sciences Center School of Nursing in Lubbock, Texas. Her research and practice as a board-certified women's health NP and OB clinical nurse specialist focus on improving the health and well-being of pregnant mothers in a medically underserved population. As a faculty member with more than 30 years of experience in teaching undergraduate and graduate nursing students and as a healthcare provider, Yondell is passionate about ensuring that students learn to provide evidence-based and individualized patient interventions.

**Carol Lynn Maxwell-Thompson, MSN, RN, FNP-C,** is an assistant professor of nursing at the University of Virginia School of Nursing. In addition to teaching and advising in the Clinical Nurse Leader Program, she is faculty advisor for the Student Nurses Association of Virginia. She has worked as an FNP at the CVS Minute Clinic and Charlottesville Free Clinic. She is an AHA BLS CPR instructor with the American Heart Association and supervises nursing students who are also AHA BLS instructors when teaching CPR classes.

**Colleen H. Meakim, MSN, RN, CHSE,** is the director of simulation and the Learning Resource Center at Villanova University. She has developed or participated in the development of many simulation scenarios and programs at Villanova. She served as a board member for 7 years for the International Nursing Association for Clinical Simulation and Learning (INACSL). She has worked and continues to work with INACSL to develop standards for key elements of simulation. She has participated in research and publications regarding simulation and debriefing methodology. She has done many presentations related to incorporating simulation into the curriculum, simulation as a teaching/learning strategy, and debriefing, and has taught a graduate course in simulation. She worked with the SSH Certification Committee from 2010 to 2014. In 2007, she received the INACSL Award for Excellence in the Academic Setting, and in 2013, she received an award for service to INACSL.

**Earline M. W. Miller, PhD, MPH, RN,** served as an associate professor of nursing at Loma Linda University School of Nursing in California. She was an instructor in pediatric nursing, and assisted with and later became the director of the Learning Assistance Program until her retirement in 2010. Previously, she taught several nursing courses at Southwestern Adventist University and community health nursing at the University of Texas in Arlington. Her clinical nursing included pediatric nursing, home health, nursing, school health nursing, and camp nursing. She appreciated The Exam Analysis© as an opportunity to encourage nursing students in their pursuit of academic success.

**Barbara L. Ninan, MN, RN,** is an assistant professor at Loma Linda University School of Nursing in California. In addition, she is an EdD student at Walden University and is anticipated to complete the doctoral program in 2015. Barbara has been the director of the Learning Assistance Program (LAP) since 2010. She worked for 35 years in the hospital setting as a clinical nurse in adult critical care, labor and delivery, postpartum, the newborn nursery, and neonatal intensive care, and then was nurse manager for labor and delivery, postpartum, and the newborn nursery. During her 20 years as nurse manager, she worked closely with the Loma Linda School of Nursing to facilitate positive experiences for nursing students in their clinical rotations in obstetrics. She also mentored nursing students during their management experience. In her current role as director of LAP, she uses The Exam Analysis$^©$ on a regular basis and is passionate about supporting the success of all nursing students and helping to prepare them as the nurses of tomorrow.

**Sharon K. Pittard, MSN, RNC,** is an associate professor at Good Samaritan College of Nursing and Health Science in Cincinnati, Ohio. She has been teaching at the college for 24 years with clinical expertise in obstetrical nursing. Sharon has designed creative and innovative teaching-learning strategies in the classroom and clinical settings.

**William Stuart Pope, DNP, RN, DMin,** is an associate clinical professor in the School of Nursing at Auburn University. His emphasis is in psychiatric nursing and communication. William is the founder and director of Canines Assisting Recovery and Education (CAREing Paws), an animal-assisted therapy program at Auburn University that focuses on working with children and adults with mental disorders in diverse settings.

**Renee T. Ridley, PhD, RN,** is a clinical associate professor in the College of Nursing at Texas A&M Health Science Center, where she teaches both BSN and MSN courses. She has been an RN since 1985, working 16 of her 30 years in the nursing profession in obstetrics and 10 years as a certified FNP. She has been involved in academia since 1990. Renee obtained her PhD from Saint Louis University in 2008, with her dissertation devoted to interactive teaching in nursing education. She has presented nationally regarding interprofessional education, as well as internationally on topics related to interactive teaching. She has published in several peer-reviewed journals and particularly enjoys co-authoring with students.

**Kelly Riley, BSN, RN,** graduated with highest honors from the University of Virginia School of Nursing. She is an RN on the acute care oncology unit at the Virginia Commonwealth University Health System, where she serves as co-chair for the Professional Practice Council, promoting evidence-based practice at the bedside, and frequently precepts new graduate RNs and nursing students.

**Keith Rischer, MA, RN, CEN, CCRN,** is an author, blogger, presenter, and recognized authority on clinical reasoning and its relevance to nursing practice, as well as a developer of creative strategies to integrate it successfully in nursing education, which are featured on his website KeithRN. In addition to 8 years of teaching both fundamental and advanced levels, he has never left clinical practice and has 31 years of experience in a wide variety of clinical settings, including critical care and the emergency department.

This combination has given Keith a unique bifocal lens to identify what is currently needed to prepare today's nurse graduates for the realities and demands of clinical practice. His work on clinical reasoning has been presented in Kozier & Erb's *Fundamentals of Nursing* and the upcoming fourth edition of *Professional Issues in Nursing: Challenges and Opportunities.*

**Mary Madeline Rogge, PhD, RN, FNP-BC,** is an associate professor at Texas Tech University Health Sciences Center School of Nursing with more than 30 years of experience in teaching in BSN, MSN, and DNP programs. She has engaged in acute and primary care. Her areas of research and scholarship primarily emphasize the pathophysiology of acute and chronic illnesses, with a special focus on obesity. She seeks to assist students in deepening their understanding of the relevance of genomics, epigenomics, and immunology in the care of patients with chronic diseases. Currently, she is developing applying informatics to the development of a taxonomy of obesity as a way to improve the diagnosis and management of this chronic disease.

**Gretchen Rosoff, MEd, RN,** is an assistant professor of nursing at Lawrence Memorial/ Regis College in Medford, Massachusetts. Her expertise is in behavioral health nursing, where she has been specializing for 41 years. She not only teaches senior nursing students to recognize and treat mental health problems but also prepares them to use human interactions to successfully negotiate the healthcare system and interact positively with collaborators, patients, and families.

**Pamela K. Rutar, EdD, MSN, RN, CNE,** is an assistant professor at Cleveland State University School of Nursing in Ohio. Her research interests include mentoring, interprofessional education, and transition to practice. Clinical interests include women's and children's health, chronic disease management, and topics related to leadership in health care, with a focus on meeting the needs of the medically underserved. Pam is an Ohio Action Coalition Task Group co-chair for transition to practice. Her experience includes more than 10 years as a nurse educator and a clinical background in women's and children's health.

**Mary Kathryn (Katie) Sanders, MSN, RN,** is a clinical assistant professor at Texas A&M University Health Science Center in Round Rock. She has more than 21 years of nursing experience in surgical, pediatric, and community health. Since obtaining her MSN in education in 2010, Katie has served as a faculty member, teaching in the traditional, second degree, and online programs. Currently, she is a DNP student at Indiana Wesleyan University, working on the linkage between caring and critical thinking.

**Jenny B. Schuessler, PhD, RN,** was appointed as a dean and professor of the Tanner Health System School of Nursing at the University of West Georgia in Carrollton in 2014. Her experience includes 14 years as an associate dean of Auburn University School of Nursing in Alabama and serves as the Betty Fuller McClendon Endowed Professor. Jenny has published extensively on curriculum development and evaluation. Her research program centers around cardiovascular nursing and care of underserved populations. Jenny's published research on heart failure has been cited in prestigious journals, such as *Archives of Internal Medicine* and *Heart and Lung*. Jenny is a leadership fellow of the American Association of Colleges of Nursing, a recipient of the American Association of Critical Care Nurses Excellence in Education Award, and a Top 100 Nursing Professor by BSN to MSN Online.

**Elaine S. Van Doren, PhD, RN,** is an associate professor at the Grand Valley State University Kirkhof College of Nursing in Grand Rapids, Michigan. During the period when the concept-based curriculum was developed and implemented, Elaine was serving as an associate dean for the undergraduate programs. In this role, she worked to provide direction for the curriculum; arranged for faculty and staff resources; and ensured follow-up for university, state, and professional requirements. With more than 27 years of academic collegiate experience, she is committed to establishing curricula that prepare nursing professionals to meet the needs of the public as described in the *Future of Nursing* report. As a past National League for Nursing Health Information Technology Scholar, she also worked to ensure the integration of informatics into the new concept-based curriculum.

**Gwyn M. Vernon, MSN, CRNP,** holds a master's degree in community health education and an MSN from the University of Pennsylvania. In 1982, Gwyn was one of the founding members of the Parkinson's Disease and Movement Disorders Center in Philadelphia, which is affiliated with the University of Pennsylvania Comprehensive Neuroscience Center and currently located at the Pennsylvania Hospital Division. Author of more than 45 peer-reviewed articles and chapters on Parkinson's disease and co-author of *Comprehensive Nursing Care for Parkinson's Disease*, she speaks nationally and internationally on the topic and is the national director of the Edmond J. Safra Visiting Nurse Faculty Program at the Parkinson's Disease Foundation. Gwyn's passion is to care for those with Parkinson's disease and to educate future generations of nurses to care for those with the disease.

**Jeanne M. Walter, PhD, RN, FAAMA,** is an assistant professor at the Virginia Commonwealth University (VCU) School of Nursing, where she serves as the director of undergraduate nursing programs. She is an experienced educator, clinician, and administrator and has been a leader in development of IPE initiatives on the health science campus of VCU, including collaborating with an IP faculty team to develop two IPE courses that are now part of the required curricula for all health science students. Jeanne has presented and published her IPE work in a number of professional venues. She is the co-principal investigator of the Art of Nursing research-teaching-learning initiative aimed at developing clinical reasoning skills in beginning nursing students.

**Patricia A. Watts, DNP, RN, CNS, PNP-BC,** is a clinical assistant professor Indiana University School of Nursing. Her NP practice is at the Bradford Woods' Residential Pediatric Camps for Children and Adolescents with Special Needs and Chronic Medical Conditions. Her research focus is maintenance of evidence-based nursing practice standards at the high-risk pediatric camps. Her DNP research resulted in successful adoption of the SBAR as the standard of camp nurse hand-off practice at the Bradford Woods' camp. Use of the Bradford Woods' pediatric camps as a clinical site for nursing and interdisciplinary healthcare students continues to be one of Patricia's major goals in education.

**Jesse S. White, BFA, MAE,** teaches visual art at John Burroughs Elementary School, a public school in Northeast Washington, DC. She builds her curriculum around close looking, solution-oriented thinking, as well as attention to detail and craft. By referring to her classroom as "the studio" and emphasizing the importance of planning and reflection, Jesse encourages her students to view themselves as artists and the art-making process as an endeavor that deserves time, energy, and brainpower. Jesse graduated summa cum laude from the University of North Carolina at Chapel Hill with a bachelor's degree in studio art and earned a master's in art education from Virginia Commonwealth University.

**Sara Wilson-McKay, PhD,** is the chair and associate professor of art education in the School of the Arts at Virginia Commonwealth University (VCU). She is the co-principal investigator of the interdisciplinary research team developing VCU's Art of Nursing. This novel art-based teaching-learning initiative brings together art education graduate students, beginning nursing students, and clinical faculty in an interprofessional relationship to address ways to enhance clinical reasoning at the bedside through rich art experiences in a museum setting. More generally, Sara's research on the politics of vision explores the ways in which works of art create new seeing, how looking can be a dialogic process, and the possibilities of seeing more of the educational process in and through art. In her publications in leading journals of art education, including *Studies in Art Education*, *Art Education*, and the *Journal of Social Theory*, Sara examines how the arts encourage democratic participation toward social action.

**Grenith J. Zimmerman, PhD,** is a professor of biostatistics at Loma Linda University. She helped to develop the research program at the School of Nursing and taught courses in research and statistics for nursing graduate and undergraduate students for several years, and she continues this relationship with consulting and data analysis for selected projects. Studying methods for enhancing student learning and understanding has been one of Grenith's lifelong interests.

# Foreword

Purpose, power, and passion give resonance to the identity of the National League for Nursing (NLN) as the voice for nursing education and as the premier organization for nurse faculty and leaders in nursing education. Our purpose is best described through our mission and core values. The NLN implements its mission—to promote excellence in nursing education to build a strong and diverse nursing workforce to advance the health of our nation and the global community—guided by four dynamic and integrated core values that permeate the organization and are reflected in its work: caring, integrity, diversity, and excellence. With the power of its 40,000 individual members and more than 1,200 member teaching institutions and healthcare organizations, the NLN boasts a remarkable past, an exceptional present, and a shared and transformative future. For more than 120 years, the NLN has had a long and celebrated history of promoting excellence in nursing education through faculty development programs, networking opportunities, testing and assessment, nursing research grants, and public policy initiatives.

With the NLN's historic move to Washington, DC, in 2013, we redesigned the NLN's organizational structure to pursue with passion the co-creation of seven Centers for Nursing Education to help nurse leaders, faculty, students, the nurse workforce, and our corporate/community partners advance the health of the nation and the global community. Not centers in the brick-and-mortar sense, they are a way of shaping our thinking and framing our work, a way to continue to lead in the areas that we believe are crucial to the future of nursing and nursing education. The NLN Centers for Nursing Education are:

- The NLN Center for Academic and Clinical Transitions
- The NLN | Chamberlain College of Nursing Center for the Advancement of the Science of Nursing Education
- The NLN Center for Assessment and Evaluation
- The NLN Center for Excellence in the Care of Vulnerable Populations
- The NLN Center for Diversity and Global Initiatives
- The NLN Center for Innovation in Simulation and Technology
- The NLN Center for Transformational Leadership

I am so pleased that Dr. Caputi, as editor of this volume, chose to arrange the chapters to correspond with the work of five of the centers—work that not only benefits nurse educators but also our students and the millions of patients for whom nurses care over the course of our professional lives. With purpose, power, and passion, the NLN centers are a resource for innovative technology for nurse educators; new models for teaching and learning, promotion, and support for the development of academic and clinical transitions; and assessment, evaluation, and development of nursing education standards. Enjoy the read.

**Beverly Malone, PhD, RN, FAAN**
CEO, NLN
May 2015

# Preface

This publication is the third in the series of books from the National League for Nursing (NLN) dedicated to Innovation in Nursing Education. The contributions of its many authors support various NLN Centers for Nursing Education. Currently, there are seven Centers for Nursing Education that focus on the important work of the NLN. The chapters in this edition specifically relate to five of those centers, which are described here. Each section of the book is devoted to one of these centers.

## THE NLN | CHAMBERLAIN COLLEGE OF NURSING CENTER FOR THE ADVANCEMENT OF THE SCIENCE OF NURSING EDUCATION (SECTION I)

The NLN recognizes that research is fundamental to quality and timely nursing education based on scientific inquiry. It is the only national nursing organization funding nursing education research. The NLN | Chamberlain College of Nursing Center for the Advancement of the Science of Nursing Education promotes evidence-based nursing education and the scholarship of teaching. The center's establishment in September 2012 began an innovative partnership to bring positive change to nursing education research for all sectors of the profession. The center supports research, develops scholarship, and produces publications that build the science of nursing education. The NLN | Chamberlain Center reaches out to partners and collaborates with research societies and organizations to sponsor programs and conferences that present and disseminate research.

## THE NLN CENTER FOR ASSESSMENT AND EVALUATION (SECTION II)

The NLN calls for multiple and fair measures for competency evaluation in nursing programs to ensure a diverse workforce. This center promotes valid, reliable, and evidence-based measurement and identifies best practices for establishing guidelines and standards of practice that recognize and value each test taker's perspective, background, and context. In addition, the center provides tools and programs for the assessment of our other centers.

## THE NLN CENTER FOR EXCELLENCE IN THE CARE OF VULNERABLE POPULATIONS (SECTION III)

The Center for Excellence in the Care of Vulnerable Populations currently addresses the special needs of older adults, veterans, Alzheimer's patients, and their caregivers. In addition, it supports the efforts of practical nursing (PN) faculty to align PN graduates with current workforce trends related to care of vulnerable populations in both acute and long-term care settings.

## THE NLN CENTER FOR TRANSFORMATIONAL LEADERSHIP (SECTION IV)

Responding to the call to integrate leadership theory across the curriculum and foster the development of leaders, the center helps nurse educators to advance through the NLN Leadership Institute. The institute is composed of three 1-year programs: LEAD, the Leadership Development Program for Simulation Educators, and the Senior Deans and Directors Leadership Program.

## THE NLN CENTER FOR INNOVATION IN SIMULATION AND TECHNOLOGY (SECTION V)

In today's technology-rich environment, nurse educators need to be up-to-date on the latest innovations in simulation, e-learning, and telehealth, as well as the integration of informatics into curricula. Known throughout the nursing education community as a staunch advocate for simulation and technology, the NLN has created simulation scenarios for use across curricula, pioneered nursing education webinars, and established an annual technology conference that is now in its second decade. Moreover, the NLN incorporates technology into all of its initiatives.

The table of contents groups the chapters by the work of the center that chapter represents. I am confident that you will enjoy reading these contributions as much as I did and that you will be able to apply the information in your daily work as you bring excellent nursing education to students all over the country and at every level of nursing. In so doing, you exemplify what the NLN is all about as the *Voice* of nursing education.

**Linda Caputi, EdD, RN, CNE, ANEF**
Professor Emerita of Nursing
College of DuPage
Glen Ellyn, Illinois
President, Linda Caputi, Inc.
Saint Charles, Illinois

# Contents

# List of Figures and Tables

# The NLN | Chamberlain College of Nursing Center for the Advancement of the Science of Nursing Education

# The Caputi Model for Teaching Thinking in Nursing

**Linda Caputi,** EdD, RN, CNE, ANEF

## INTRODUCTION

*Critical thinking* is a term that has been used in nursing education for decades. Students must learn to think critically. Critical thinking in nursing is often identified with other terms, such as nursing judgment, clinical judgment, and clinical reasoning. Whatever term a nursing program uses, it is important that the term is defined and the teaching of thinking is taught in a systematic, organized manner across the curriculum.

Nursing programs create amazing curricula that offer a systematic approach to their delivery. Pre-licensure nursing programs are planned using the familiar simple-to-complex structure. Simple content is taught at the beginning, with increasingly complex content taught during subsequent academic terms. Theory content is carefully planned across the curriculum, ensuring that students have a basic knowledge base on which to build more complex content.

Psychomotor skills are also taught using the simple-to-complex approach. For example, students first learn to administer oral medications, then parenteral medications, culminating in intravenous medications requiring complex calculations based on body weight or other metrics. Each psychomotor skill is explained in a step-by-step fashion.

This approach to curriculum unpacks the vast amount of content and psychomotor skills to enable students to learn pieces of the curriculum in an organized manner. The curriculum expands on the pieces to form a whole, coalescing all content by the end of the curriculum.

Careful planning of the curriculum ensures the best learning results. Students in a pre-licensure nursing program are unfamiliar with nursing, what nurses know, and what nurses do. Therefore, the vast array of information is carefully chosen and meticulously planned as students work through the curriculum. This vast knowledge base of nursing content and psychomotor skills are "unpacked," presenting the basic building blocks first and then expanding on the knowledge base as the student progresses.

Interestingly, this type of painstaking attention to the unpacking, teaching, and expanding, culminating in the education of a nurse, is not always applied to the teaching of thinking. This chapter offers thoughts about how the teaching of thinking may be unpacked for students as they learn the building blocks of clinical reasoning.

## FROM A STUDENT'S PERSPECTIVE

Students often do not consider the importance of learning and applying thinking. Many faculty still complain that students in theory sessions just want to know what they will need to know for the test. When learning in the clinical setting, students desire to perform as many psychomotor skills as possible. They may believe that the more psychomotor skills they perform, the more they are learning to be a nurse. Students often times do not appreciate the importance of spending time in the clinical engaging in critical thinking and clinical reasoning activities when instead they could spend the time performing psychomotor skills.

Students want to be nurses. They see what nurses do and hear what nurses say about medical diagnoses and how to care for patients from the medical model perspective. However, they do not hear, nor do they see, how nurses engage in thinking. Nurses think through and solve hundreds of problems every day. Many of the problems solved by nurses relate to patient care. However, many other problems solved relate to the healthcare environment, interactions with other healthcare providers, constant interruptions, and a host of other issues. Because students cannot see the mental processes in which nurses engage in a constant manner throughout the day, they may not understand the importance of how complicated these thinking processes can be.

Nursing faculty have the responsibility to uncover and unpack the thinking processes used by nurses. Faculty can do this by using a systematic, formalized approach to teach thinking across the curriculum. Critical thinking must be uncovered and overt through specific language that is deliberately taught and used if it is to be valued (Rubenfeld & Scheffer, 2015). Many times, faculty ask students to use critical thinking or to explain their thinking. Students attempt to speak to the faculty's request without actually knowing how to think, mainly because they did not learn how to think in nursing situations. They have not learned specific thinking processes (or may have learned them but not applied them in structured learning situations) to enable them to articulate their thinking.

## THREE COMPONENTS OF TEACHING CRITICAL THINKING/CLINICAL REASONING

The unpacking process begins with identifying the components of clinical reasoning. The Caputi model for teaching thinking in nursing, developed in 2011 after years of studying the literature on thinking in nursing, presents an approach for teaching clinical reasoning using specific language that unpacks and uncovers thinking. Students are taught and learn to use this language as they approach problem solving in all learning environments. The three components are:

- Benner's novice to expert theory (Benner, 2001)
- Tanner's clinical reasoning model (Tanner, 2006)
- Critical thinking skills and strategies

These components come together to provide a structure to teach critical thinking/clinical reasoning.

# Component 1: Benner's Novice to Expert Theory

The first component is derived from Benner's application of the Dreyfus model of skill acquisition (Dreyfus & Dreyfus, 1986), first published in 1984, to nursing. This groundbreaking work describes the stages of developing nurses as they become experts in their practice. Benner's model covers five stages. Two of those stages are pertinent to pre-license nursing education.

When students enter a nursing program, they are considered to be in the novice stage. They arrive with no experience of nursing situations at the scope of practice they are studying. Faculty deconstruct the nursing content by putting it into simpler, out-of-context terms so that this new learner can understand what is being taught. The novice learns specific rules to follow and applies them to all situations, regardless of context. Their practice is based on rules.

Faculty often share with students at this level that nursing is not black or white, but grey. Faculty must explain what is meant by *grey*. Grey really means "it depends." The "it depends" answer requires situational thinking, not rule-based thinking. During the first semester of nursing courses, faculty must demonstrate to students how the rules they are learning are applied to a patient considering all aspects of the patient's situation. Then the nurse can make a decision. Simply applying a rule to all situations without considering the context of the patient will lead to faulty thinking and poor decisions.

Once students have learned the "grey" lesson and have practiced applying rules within a patient context, they are ready to be guided into the advanced beginner stage of Benner's skills acquisition model. In this stage, the student is provided additional experiences with using rules in real and/or simulated situations to move from simple rules to guide behavior to applying principles to guide actions. Students are provided practice applying rules and learning about aspects of a situation that are relevant, as well as aspects of a situation that are not relevant, based on the specific patient situation. As students engage in these types of experiences, they begin to use clinical reasoning based on the specifics of a situation—that is, decisions made and actions taken become situation driven rather than rule driven.

At this point, faculty build on these experiences by planning activities that provide opportunities for students to apply rules to individual patient situations. Students compare and contrast patients with similar conditions to discover the individual patient nuances that result in situational thinking rather than rule-based thinking. Thus, students begin to learn differences among patients who appear similar but are quite different based on patient context.

A curriculum that provides a formalized, systematic approach to teaching thinking enables students to enter the advanced beginner stage in the second semester of clinical nursing courses. This type of thinking is used throughout the remainder of the program and introduces increasingly complex situations.

# Component 2: Tanner's Clinical Reasoning Model

The second component, Tanner's clinical reasoning model (Tanner, 2006), uses four steps:

1. Noticing
2. Interpreting

3. Responding

4. Reflecting

Faculty can turn these four steps into specific questions for students:

1. What did you notice?

2. What does it mean?

3. What will you do?

4. What was the effect of what you did?

Using these four questions provides students with a framework for organizing their overall thinking about a situation.

To further guide students' use of this model, faculty can consider their role in helping the student apply the model. These four steps are now reworded, presenting the active role of faculty in guiding students:

1. *Noticing:* Faculty focus students' "perceptual awareness" as the first step.

2. *Interpreting:* Faculty then guide students' noticing of a situation to interpret the situation correctly, applying critical thinking skills.

3. *Responding:* Faculty help students determine how to respond in the context of a specific patient.

4. *Reflecting:* Faculty ask students to immediately reflect on what was just done, learn from it, correct their thinking, and then use what they learned in the next similar situation.

## Component 3: Critical Thinking Skills and Strategies

The third component is a listing of specific critical thinking skills and strategies. Breaking down critical thinking into its parts means teaching students *specific* critical thinking skills and strategies. This is often the critical piece missing when faculty ask students to explain their thinking (Caputi, 2010a, 2010b). Faculty ask students questions such as:

• What is the basis for your decision?

• What decision did you make and why?

• What will you do next and why?

Even students who know the correct answer about what they will do for the patient may not be able to explain their thinking. This may occur not because they do not know how to think, but rather because they have never had thinking put into concrete terms, so they cannot track or explain their thinking. They may have discovered the answer to the question using critical thinking but cannot articulate how they arrived at the answer because they have not specifically learned thinking skills and strategies used to arrive at the answer. They do not have the knowledge base related to thinking skills that is needed to answer that question. Students often struggle because they have not learned what faculty *mean* by thinking. Frustrated, students often ask themselves the following questions:

- How do I answer the "why" question?
- When did I learn to answer why questions?
- Where do I begin?
- How do I organize my thoughts?
- Just what does the teacher mean? I have no idea!!!

Without having a knowledge base about thinking, students are not able to apply metacognition, which is what faculty are asking students to do with the why questions. Metacognition refers to thinking about one's thinking. Metacognition refers to students' ability to understand their thinking and control their cognitive processes. Specific learning about cognitive processes is often lacking in formal nursing education, which may be why students struggle to answer the why questions.

Nurses use many critical thinking skills and strategies. These thinking skills are critical for students to learn so that they can explain their thinking and apply metacognition—thinking about their thinking. This critical piece is often missing in teaching students to think like a nurse. Students often receive a list of these thinking skills and even definitions, but that is not enough. They need specific guidance in applying thinking skills in clinical situations. Throughout the nursing education literature, there are approximately 18 critical thinking skills (Alfaro-LeFevre, 2013; Caputi, 2010a, 2010b; Paul & Elder, 2014). Following is a brief list that is not all inclusive; there are others:

- Analyzing data
- Judging how much ambiguity is acceptable
- Setting priorities
- Determining the importance of information
- Predicting and managing potential complications
- Distinguishing relevant from irrelevant information for THIS patient

Students not only must learn what these are but also must *use* them in the clinical situation. It is best to ensure that this is done in the first clinical course. Through this process, students learn what is meant by "nursing is not black or white, but grey." The next section presents an example.

## TEACHING THE THINKING SKILL OF HOW MUCH AMBIGUITY CAN BE TOLERATED IN A PATIENT SITUATION

In the beginning nursing course, students learn the psychomotor skill of taking vital signs. They learn the "within normal limits" rules of vital signs. It is critical for nurses to decide how much ambiguity can be tolerated for an individual patient from the within normal limits of vital signs. Students can learn how to use this thinking skill in the first nursing course.

The faculty teaches the skill of deciding how much ambiguity can be tolerated in a situation. Using this skill, the situation is considered and a rule applied, not in a strict sense but in "how much wiggle room" can be tolerated when applying the rule.

As faculty teach the thinking skill during class, an everyday life example is provided. The faculty might share that when driving a car and merging onto an expressway, a rule is considered. That rule is the speed limit, considering the maximum and minimum posted limits. However, before deciding the wiggle room when considering the actual rate of speed that will be driven, the driver collects data. That data may include:

- Amount of traffic
- Weather conditions
- Condition of the road
- Where the police officers may be
- Number of traffic violations of the driver

After quickly considering all data, the driver makes a decision about what speed above the posted limit can be safely driven, if weather and road conditions are favorable. Or, if the data reveal issues with weather or road conditions, how much slower to drive than the posted minimum.

This same kind of thinking is applied to vital signs. That week when students attend clinical, two students will engage in a clinical reasoning activity to apply the thinking skill of how much ambiguity can be tolerated in a patient situation. These two students take vital signs on three patients for whom other students are caring. They then complete the tool presented in Box 1.1.

The purpose of this activity is to teach how nurses think through a specific patient situation—that is, how to apply a specific thinking skill. They must collect data, analyze the data, and determine the importance of information, all within the context of the patient, before they can determine how to apply the rules they learned about within normal limits for vital signs.

During postconference, the faculty help students process this information as they work to the final goal of determining how much ambiguity can be tolerated in a patient situation. The two students present each patient, one at a time. They sort through all assessment data, then consider what they learned about the patient's pathology, pre-existing conditions, level of pain, and so forth. The faculty then help students consider all data as they make decisions about the vital signs. Students then look at the second and third patients. Once finished making a decision about each patient's vital signs, the faculty help them compare and contrast. Why was a blood pressure acceptable for one patient but perhaps not for the other? The faculty then help students think through the skill of applying parameters as they engage in clinical forethought determining what vital sign readings would trigger action by the nurse and what actions the nurse would take.

The purpose of the assignment is not to teach students a list of steps to memorize when considering a patient's vital signs. The purpose is to provide an actual patient situation where a specific critical thinking skill is applied to arrive at a decision based on the situation or the context of the patient. Once students have worked through this assignment, in subsequent clinical sessions students will report the patient's vital signs and their thinking as applied in this situation.

The ultimate goal is for students to apply this thinking to other decisions regarding individual patients. It is this thinking process that is expected when answering the why

## BOX 1.1

# Judging How Much Ambiguity Can Be Tolerated Vital Signs Activity

For each of 3 patients, complete the following.

Age:                    Gender:

Current:

    Blood Pressure:

    Pulse:

    Temperature:

    Respirations:

Last 24 hours vital signs:

Normal vital signs for this patient:

Activity level:

Medical diagnosis:

Preexisting conditions:

Pain rating:

Medications (complete the following for all medications this patient is currently taking):

    Name:

    Classification:

    Effect on any of the vital signs:

Procedures/treatments performed:

Effect of procedures/treatments on any of the vital signs:

**Process the Information in Postconference**
- Help students compare the 3 patients.
- Determine why vital signs acceptable for one patient may not be acceptable for one of the other patients.
- Help them establish parameters and discuss what to do if the patient's vital signs go outside the parameters—establishing clinical forethought.

questions. Therefore, the follow-up expectation is for students to reply about any patient data in the following manner:

- What are your assessment data?
- What data are out of range?
- What further data did/should you collect?
- What will you do with that data?

- How will you use that additional data to make a decision about the original assessment data?
- What parameters will you apply that will call you to action?

When students can explain their thinking, they are better able to answer the why questions presented earlier:

- What is the basis for your decision?
- What decision did you make and why?
- What will you do next and why?

This is one example of applying one critical thinking skill. For every critical thinking skill taught in the first semester of a nursing course, a clinical application is provided. In this manner, students learn to use critical thinking skills, thus gaining insight into how to answer the why questions by basing their answers on the application of actual thinking processes. As students progress through the nursing courses, they continue to apply these thinking processes to increasingly complex situations.

## PUTTING THE THREE COMPONENTS TOGETHER

None of the individual components alone can result in learning how to think like a nurse. They all work together to build thinking across the curriculum. Faculty ask questions related to the four steps of Tanner's clinical reasoning model. The student must use critical thinking skills when working through each step of Tanner's model. For example, a student is caring for a patient who is 2 days post abdominal surgery necessitated by a ruptured appendix. The student states that the patient has abdominal pain and is requesting simethicone (Gas-X). The faculty asks the student to apply Tanner's clinical reasoning model and identify critical thinking skills as the student thinks through the situation. Box 1.2 presents the student's thinking.

As students become skilled using thinking skills by applying Tanner's model and specific thinking skills, they move through Benner's novice stage and enter the advanced beginner stage. The very deliberate assignments that expose students to individual patient situations that influence the way in which the data are interpreted moves them from novice to advanced beginner. They move from rule-based thinking into the stage of situation-based thinking.

## MOVING THROUGH BENNER'S FINAL THREE STAGES OF SKILL ACQUISITION

Students need an organized approach to learning when they enter a nursing program. Nursing is new and even foreign to them. Faculty design a curriculum that proceeds from simple to complex, leveling content and nursing skills across the program. Initial learning is structured with simple relationships among concepts in theory and step-by-step guidelines for nursing skills. As students advance through the program, their performance of nursing skills and application of nursing knowledge becomes less rule based and more situational. This becomes obvious when students no longer need an extended amount of time to take a set of vital signs compared to the length of time required in

**BOX 1.2**

## Applying the Four Questions of Tanner's Clinical Reasoning Model

### Question #1: What did I notice?
- The patient is 4 days postop following abdominal surgery.
- On IV antibiotics due to preoperative leakage of infection into the peritoneal cavity.
- Currently reports "gas" pains and requests simethicone.
- Bowel sounds present but hypoactive.

**CT skills used:** Identifying signs and symptoms; predicting and managing potential complications; gathering complete and accurate data; determining the importance of information

### Question #2: What does it mean?
Trapped gas in a sluggish colon OR possible complication developing: paralytic ileus

**CT skills used:** Analysis of data

### Question #3: What will I do?
I will consider both my answers to "What does it mean?" when determining actions to take.

1. I can give the requested simethicone
   or I can first:
2. Investigate further:
   a. Is the patient taking narcotics? How much; how often?
   b. Did the patient have anything else done today for this concern?
   c. Is the patient taking in enough fluids to prevent constipation?
   d. Is the patient ambulating?
   e. Does the patient have bowel sounds in all four quadrants?
3. Based on the answers to these questions:
   a. Give the simethicone
   b. Monitor the IV fluids the patient is receiving to ensure the patient is hydrated
   c. Ambulate the patient more often
   d. Continue to auscultate bowel sounds every 8 hours

**CT skills used:** Setting priorities

### Question #4: What was the effect of what I did?
To be determined with follow-up assessments.

their initial learning. The student's performance of nursing skills and application of theory become less deliberate and more automatic as they move through the program.

This is the goal with teaching thinking. In the initial phases, students learn all three major components of the Caputi model for teaching thinking in nursing, as well as all aspects related to each of these three components. As they apply their learning in clinical practice, thinking should become automatic rather than a deliberate step-by-step process. However, before automaticity becomes possible, students must learn the thinking skills and strategies. Without learning the building blocks of thinking in nursing, they cannot think about their thinking but only hope that their thinking is correct as they work to answer the why questions posed.

## SUMMARY

The Caputi model for teaching thinking in nursing is fairly simple and can be summarized as follows:

1. Teach individual critical thinking skills.

2. Give students deliberate, focused practice applying each of the thinking skills in either an actual patient or classroom patient situation.

3. Demonstrate how what they are doing aligns with Tanner's evidence-based model of clinical reasoning.

4. Demonstrate how they are progressing through the thinking of Benner's stages of novice and advanced beginner.

5. Continue this process across your curriculum.

6. Create a critical thinking curriculum!!

The end goal for implementing a deliberate approach to teaching thinking is improved patient outcomes. When new graduates apply for their first nursing position, they must talk this talk. As they share with their interviewer all of the psychomotor skills they performed while in the clinical setting throughout school, they should also share all of the specific thinking skills they learned and how they applied them to identify potential complications, decrease the morbidity and mortality rate, and decrease the failure to rescue rate. When students can articulate these learned thinking skills for the purpose of improving patient care, then we have performed a job well done.

### References

Alfaro-LeFevre, R. (2013). *Critical thinking, clinical reasoning, and clinical judgment: A practical approach.* St. Louis, MO: Elsevier.

Benner, P. (2001). *From novice to expert: Excellence and power in clinical nursing practice.* (Commemorative edition). Upper Saddle River, NJ: Prentice Hall.

Caputi, L. (2010a). An introduction to developing critical thinking in nursing education. In L. Caputi (Ed.), *Teaching nursing: The art and science* (vol. 2, pp. 381–390). Glen Ellyn, IL: DuPage Press.

Caputi, L. (2010b). Operationalizing critical thinking. In L. Caputi (Ed.), *Teaching nursing: The art and science* (vol. 2, pp. 391–412). Glen Ellyn, IL: DuPage Press.

Dreyfus, H. L., & Dreyfus, S. E. (1986). *Mind over machine: The power of human intuition and expertise in the era of the computer.* New York, NY: Free Press.

Paul, R., & Elder, L. (2014). *The miniature guide to critical thinking: Concepts and tools* (7th ed.). Dillon Beach, CA: Foundation for Critical Thinking.

Rubenfeld, M. G., & Scheffer, B. K. (2015). *Critical thinking TACTICS for nurses: Achieving the IOM competencies* (3rd ed.). Sudbury, MA: Jones & Bartlett.

Tanner, C. (2006). Thinking like a nurse: A research-based model of clinical judgment in nursing. *Journal of Nursing Education, 45*(6), 204–211.

# 2

# Why Clinical Reasoning Is Foundational to Nursing Practice

**Keith Rischer,** MA, RN, CEN, CCRN

The research findings of the Carnegie Foundation have made it clear that nursing education is in need of radical transformation because the current structure of nursing education is not adequate to prepare students for clinical practice. To be prepared for clinical practice and think like a nurse, students must understand and then incorporate clinical reasoning into their practice (Benner, Sutphen, Leonard, & Day, 2010). Therefore, it is the responsibility of nurse educators to ensure that every student has clinical reasoning skills before graduation (Jensen, 2013). Clinical reasoning is the ability of the nurse to think in action and reason as a situation changes, recognizing and then responding appropriately to a patient's deteriorating condition (Benner et al., 2010).

When nurses are unable to clinically reason by recognizing a change in status before it is too late, patients die, and those deaths could be prevented if not for the failure to "rescue" by the nurse (Clarke & Aiken, 2003). The correlation and connection between patient safety and clinical reasoning and the resultant impact on patient care delivered by the now autonomous graduate nurses must guide curriculum development, integration, and leveling of clinical reasoning in nursing education.

## CLINICAL REASONING DEFINED

Student understanding and use of clinical reasoning skills must be emphasized and leveled in nursing education. Clinical reasoning involves the complex processes a nurse uses to make clinical judgments by selecting from alternatives, weighing the evidence, and using intuition and pattern recognition (Tanner, 2006). It is also a logical process by which nurses collect cues, process the information, understand the patient problem, plan and implement interventions, evaluate outcomes, and reflect on and learn from the process (Levett-Jones et al., 2010). There is no substitute for clinical experience to strengthen and develop clinical reasoning. Experienced nurses are more proficient than new graduates in predicting or anticipating patient problems and proactively practice by collecting data to identify and prevent patient complications. In contrast, novice nurses tend to practice reactively, searching for cues after a problem is identified (Levett-Jones et al., 2010). Novice student nurses with limited clinical experience are particularly vulnerable to failure to rescue (Clarke & Aiken, 2003).

Because of a lack of clinical experience and lack of context, novice nurses tend to be concrete, textbook learners (Benner, 1984). Clinical reasoning must first be concretely and succinctly defined before students can grasp, understand, and apply clinical reasoning to clinical practice. A practical, working definition that captures the essence of clinical reasoning to nursing practice is found in the work of Patricia Benner. She describes clinical reasoning as the ability of the nurse to think in action and reason as a situation changes over time by capturing and understanding the significance of clinical trajectories (Benner et al., 2010). She and her colleagues later defined it as the ability to focus and filter clinical data in order to recognize what is most and least important so the nurse can identify if an actual problem is present (Benner, Hooper-Kyriakidis, & Stannard, 2011).

Derived from this definition of clinical reasoning are four primary components of clinical reasoning:

1. Think in action and reason as a situation changes
2. Identify which clinical data are relevant
3. Understand the significance of clinical trends of relevant data
4. Make a clinical judgment to determine if an actual problem is present

Each component of this definition can be used to guide student understanding and application to clinical practice to establish the knowledge base needed to clinically reason in practice.

## Component 1: Think in Action and Reason as a Situation Changes

Patients do not typically stay static over time; they either improve or gradually or quickly deteriorate. Just as a lifeguard continually and vigilantly scans the water for signs of a struggling swimmer, to rescue a patient from a deteriorating change of status, the nurse must also be vigilant to determine if the patient may be developing a change in status by using the thinking skill of clinical reasoning. A key component of clinical reasoning is the ability to think in action (Benner et al., 2010). Therefore, students must be prepared to think on their feet and recognize the nursing priority when the status of patients change and be skilled in early recognition and management if a change in status occurs (Shoulders, Follett, & Eason, 2014).

In addition to thinking in action, the nurse must also anticipate the most likely or worst possible complications for each patient in his or her care (Rischer, 2013). Doing so develops the skill of being proactive in clinical practice. A problem must first be anticipated and then recognized when it occurs before the nurse can intervene and do something about the problem (del Bueno, 2005). Once a life-threatening complication begins to develop, it is the responsibility of the nurse to identify the problem early and take control by implementing appropriate interventions. The primary reasons complications progress include failure by the nurse to anticipate the problem, failure to recognize its presence when it develops, failure to initiate appropriate nursing interventions, and inappropriate management of the complication (Clarke & Aiken, 2003).

## Component 2: Identify Which Clinical Data Are Relevant

The growing amount of information that students are expected to master in nursing education is a barrier to student learning and mastery of content (del Bueno, 2005). Nursing curricula tend to be additive over time. Rather than removing and reworking current content, faculty often add more (Benner et al., 2010; Tanner, 2004). Benner (1984) identified that a characteristic of novice student nurses is that all content is seen as relevant, and as a result, they are unable to differentiate what is most and least important to clinical practice. This lack of ability to differentiate among data adversely impacts mastery because students obtain a superficial learning of a broad amount of subject matter but lack the deep learning of what is most important to practice.

To develop a sense of salience and identify what clinical data are most relevant, students must develop a deep understanding of the applied sciences, including areas such as pathophysiology, fluids and electrolytes, and a host of other related information. Students must be able to contextualize their understanding of this scientific material to the care of the individual patient. It is only when deep knowledge of the most important content has been understood that the student is able to apply, analyze, and see the relevance of clinical data in the context of patient care (Olson, 2000).

Relevant clinical data are identified through knowledge of the applied sciences. This knowledge is applied in the clinical setting when analyzing physical assessment findings, vital signs, and laboratory values. For example, for a patient with heart failure, the following clinical data are collected and identified as relevant:

- 2+ pitting edema in lower legs
- Coarse bibasilar crackles
- Respiratory rate 24/minute with $O_2$ sat 88 percent on room air
- BP: 178/88
- Creatinine: 1.9 mg/dL; last creatinine was 1.1 mg/dL
- BNP: 1125 ng/L; last BNP was 210 ng/L

Once clinical data are correctly identified as relevant, the next step of clinical reasoning is to trend this data to determine the clinical trajectory (Benner et al., 2010).

## Component 3: Understand the Significance of Clinical Trends of Relevant Data

Identifying and trending the most important or relevant clinical data by comparing current data to previous readings is an essential component of clinical reasoning and a hallmark of thinking like a nurse (Benner et al., 2010). To rescue a patient with a change in status, the nurse must be able to recognize subtle changes in the patient's condition over time. Rescue is facilitated when the nurse trends relevant clinical data and intentionally assesses early manifestations of the most likely or worst possible complication. The early, subtle changes in a patient's status must be recognized before a problem progresses and results in an adverse outcome. In addition to trending vital signs and nursing assessment data, relevant laboratory values and outcomes of previous nursing interventions must be trended as well.

Review the same example of relevant clinical data that was identified in a patient with heart failure:

- 2+ pitting edema in lower legs
- Coarse bibasilar crackles
- Respiratory rate 24/minute with $O_2$ sat 88 percent on room air
- BP: 178/88
- Creatinine: 1.9 mg/dL; last creatinine was 1.1 mg/dL
- BNP: 1125 ng/L; last BNP was 210 ng/L

Each aspect of this clinical data can and must be trended from the onset to the most recent values. Based on the relevant laboratory values of creatinine trending from 1.1 to now 1.9 mg/dL, and the BNP trend that has increased from 210 to 1125 ng/L, when knowledge from the applied sciences is deeply understood, it becomes readily apparent that these laboratory trends reveal a worsening in both renal function and decompensation of underlying heart failure. This knowledge guides the nurse to clinically reason and then make a correct clinical judgment by connecting scientific understandings to the physical assessment findings.

## Component 4: Make a Clinical Judgment to Determine if an Actual Problem Is Present

If a nurse in practice is unable to clinically reason, the results can be an incorrect clinical judgment. To consistently formulate safe and correct clinical judgments, the nurse must be able to use knowledge, integrate nursing process, think critically, and use clinical reasoning to make a correct clinical judgment (Alfaro-Lefevre, 2013). Clinical reasoning describes the way nurses reflectively think about their thinking, use nursing knowledge to quickly review and analyze clinical data, evaluate the relevance of this clinical data, then formulate a judgment that leads to action (Koharchik, Caputi, Robb, & Culleiton, 2015).

Clinical judgment is the end result and hallmark of professional practice. Clinical judgment can be defined as the interpretation or conclusion about what a patient needs and/or the decision to take action or not (Tanner, 2006). To make a correct clinical judgment, clinical reasoning is used to:

- Select from all alternatives
- Understand the rationale for each alternative
- Collect and recognize the significance of clinical data
- Process this information to understand the current problem
- Identify the current care priority and plan of care (Levett-Jones et al., 2010)

## HOW THE "WHAT" DEVELOPS CLINICAL REASONING

To strengthen the ability of nurses to make a correct clinical judgment, the most effective intervention identified in the research of del Bueno [2005] was to have nurses work with a preceptor who would coach new nurses by repeatedly asking questions, such as "What evidence do you have or need to collect to determine the effectiveness of your intervention?" (p. 282). Asking questions is an effective strategy to develop the critical and clinical thinking that is required for practice.

The author has developed a series of questions that are relevant to ask students during medication administration that involve asking the "what":

- What is the pharmacologic class?
- What is the mechanism of action (in your own words)?
- What is the expected patient response based on the mechanism of action?
- What assessment data do you need to consider before administering the medication and to collect regarding the effectiveness of the medication?

When students can verbalize this series of what questions, they have communicated that they have the necessary foundational knowledge and are safe to administer the medication (Rischer, 2013).

## "WHAT IF"

The what series of questions guides students to identify the most likely/worst possible complication. This is the first step to prepare students to rescue if there is a change in status. In the clinical setting, faculty can use the most common complications in their specific setting to help develop this proactive nurse thinking skill. Expect students to not only identify the nursing assessments but also the interventions if any of these complications develop.

The following are examples of this line of questioning (Rischer, 2013):
*"What if" your patient …*

- Develops chest pain?
- Develops a temp of 101?
- Experiences a drop in BP to 90/50?
- Develops acute confusion on patient-controlled analgesia?
- Develops a rapid irregular heart rate of 140?
- Develops sudden onset of shortness of breath?

## HOW THE "WHY" DEVELOPS CLINICAL REASONING

To assess and evaluate the thinking and the depth of student mastery of essential content that is foundational to clinical reasoning, there is one short question that can be asked in the classroom, simulation lab, and clinical settings. Ask each student "why?" regarding everything the nurse does in practice. Students must be able to understand and answer the rationale or why of everything done in the clinical setting. As a clinical instructor, I routinely ask each of my students the following why questions:

- Why will you straight catheterize a patient post-op who has been unable to void for the past 6 hours?

- Why will you administer morphine 2 mg IV prn and not Norco prn?
- Why will you encourage your post-op patient to use the incentive spirometer every 1 to 2 hours while awake?

Am I just antagonizing my students, or do I have a reason for asking each of these why questions? Understanding the why is the foundation for safe patient care. It is only when each student has a deep understanding of the rationale for every intervention in practice that the student can be considered safe. If a new order or medication does not make sense based on the student's understanding or rationale, it must be questioned and not followed blindly. Students must be encouraged to recognize that they have a responsibility to develop their knowledge base for the purpose of developing this sense of salience and understanding the rationale for all activities performed in clinical practice. When the scientific rationale or why is understood and integrated with all that a nurse does in practice, the big picture is understood and clinical reasoning is realized (Gonzol & Newby, 2013).

Asking students to state their rationale for everything that is done in practice is also an effective way to check for faulty assumptions or a mistaken grasp of the current clinical situation. Verbalizing rationales is an important step in internalizing this aspect of clinical reasoning in practice (Benner et al., 2010). A major aspect of clinical reasoning is being able to state and understand the rationale for what is done in practice (Levett-Jones et al., 2010).

del Bueno (2005) identified a relationship between the inability of a nurse to state the correct rationale and make a correct clinical judgment. Her work focused on the ability of graduate nurses to make basic clinical judgments to recognize a problem, then correctly state the rationale or the why for essential interventions. Based on her research, only 35 percent of new RN graduates met entry-level expectations for clinical judgment. An inability to support nursing actions with correct rationale appeared to be a contributing factor. del Bueno (2005) provides the following misunderstandings of new graduates as examples of faulty thinking:

- Give heparin as an anticoagulant to trick the body and stop the bleeding
- Strain the urine for size and number of ketones (DKA)
- Give oxygen to perfuse the kidneys
- Give IV fluids with Lasix for hypovolemic shock to replace lost fluids but not raise BP
- Give D50 bolus to bring blood sugar down when it was already 620

As demonstrated with the preceding examples, these newly graduated nurses provided incorrect rationales.

## CONCLUSION

To prepare students for the current demands of clinical practice, nursing education must emphasize clinical reasoning. Clinical reasoning is an essential thinking skill that makes it possible for the nurse to make a correct clinical judgment. This will translate to improved patient outcomes and prevent patient deaths due to failure to rescue when an unidentified complication progresses. Faculty can assist students in developing clinical reasoning by posing a series of questions that emphasize applying knowledge to patient care and identifying the rationale for all that is done in practice. Because clinical reasoning is essential to safe nursing practice, it is the responsibility of nurse educators to ensure that each student demonstrates achievement of clinical reasoning prior to graduation for the purpose of providing safe, quality care resulting in improved patient outcomes.

## References

Alfaro-LeFevre, R. (2013). *Critical thinking, clinical reasoning, and clinical judgment: A practical approach* (5th ed.). St. Louis, MO: Elsevier.

Benner, P. (1984). *From novice to expert: Excellence and power in clinical nursing practice.* Upper Saddle River, NJ: Prentice Hall.

Benner, P., Hooper-Kyriakidis, P., & Stannard, D. (2011). *Clinical wisdom and interventions in acute and critical care: A thinking-in-action approach.* (2nd ed.). New York, NY: Springer.

Benner, P., Sutphen, M., Leonard, V., & Day, L. (2010). *Educating nurses: A call for radical transformation.* San Francisco, CA: Jossey-Bass.

Clarke, S. P., & Aiken, L. H. (2003). Failure to rescue. *American Journal of Nursing, 103*(1), 42–47.

del Bueno, D. (2005). A crisis in critical thinking. *Nursing Education Perspectives, 26*(5), 278–282.

Gonzol, K., & Newby, C. (2013). Facilitating clinical reasoning in the skills laboratory: Reasoning model versus nursing process-based skills checklist. *Nursing Education Perspectives, 34*(4), 265–267.

Jensen, R. (2013). Clinical reasoning during simulation: Comparison of student and faculty ratings. *Nurse Education in Practice, 13*(1), 23–28.

Koharchik, L., Caputi, L., Robb, M., & Culleiton, A. L. (2015). Fostering clinical reasoning in nursing students. *American Journal of Nursing, 115*(1), 58–61.

Levett-Jones, T., Hoffman, K., Dempsey, J., Yeun-Sim Jeong, S., Noble, D., Norton, C., et al. (2010). The 'five rights' of clinical reasoning: An educational model to enhance nursing students' ability to identify and manage clinically 'at risk' patients. *Nurse Education Today, 30*(6), 515–520.

Olson, I. (2000). *The arts and critical thinking in American education.* Stamford, CT: Bergin & Garvey.

Rischer, K. (2013). *eBook: Think like a nurse! Practical preparation for professional practice.* Available from KeithRN Web site, http://www.keithrn.com/product/ebook-think-like-a-nurse-practical-preparation-for-professional-practice/

Shoulders, B., Follett, C., & Eason, J. (2014). Enhancing critical thinking in clinical practice. *Dimensions in Critical Care Nursing, 33*(4), 207–214.

Tanner, C. A. (2004). The meaning of curriculum: Content to be covered or stories to be heard? *Journal of Nursing Education, 43*(1), 3–4.

Tanner, C. A. (2006). Thinking like a nurse: A research-based model of clinical judgment in nursing. *Journal of Nursing Education, 45*(6), 204–211.

# 3

# So, How DID You Do That? One College's Process for Creating and Implementing a Concept-Based Curriculum

**Deborah R. Bambini,** PhD, WHNP-BC, CNE, CHSE, ANEF

**Elaine S. Van Doren,** PhD, RN

Curricular change is a daunting prospect for most nursing faculty. However, content saturation, the increasing complexity of health care, and a renewed emphasis on quality and safety demand change. Many nursing programs are moving toward a concept-based approach, but few have completed the process and/or have written about it. While there cannot, and should not, be a cookie-cutter plan for undergoing such a process, examples from those who have gone through the change can be valuable to others. This chapter explains the process the faculty in one college of nursing used to implement a major curricular change that resulted in a concept-based curriculum. This change was developed for a baccalaureate program with an annual enrollment of 400 students in a mid-size midwestern university. The authors identified six stages that occurred during the process of curriculum revision:

1. Awakening
2. Exploring
3. Preparing
4. Designing
5. Implementing
6. Evaluating

Details within each of these stages are presented in this chapter.

## STEP 1: AWAKENING

*Awakening* describes the stage of becoming aware of the need for change. Awakening occurred subtly over a number of years. National reports (Institute of Medicine, 2000, 2003; QSEN Institute, 2007; Technology Informatics Guiding Education Reform [TIGER], 2006), *Educating*

**21**

*Nurses: A Call for Radical Transformation* (Benner, Stuphen, Leonard, & Day, 2010), and workshops led by nursing education experts have all contributed to the increased cognizance of the need for change. Additional factors affecting the curriculum (content saturation, challenges for clinical placement sites, and philosophy and framework revisions) supported the need for retooling the way nursing education was offered. The faculty performed an analysis of the strengths, weaknesses, opportunities, and threats (SWOT) to identify issues while acknowledging and honoring the best parts of the existing curriculum. This approach resulted in a buy-in from the majority of faculty. Awakening occurred when the following questions were asked:

1. What is the status of our undergraduate program?
2. In what ways are health care and the nursing profession developing?
3. How do we best implement the recommendations developing at the national level?

## STEP 2: EXPLORING

Once the awakening phase occurred for a critical mass of faculty, the Curriculum Revision Task Force (CRTF) was created, marking the beginning of the *exploring* phase. The CRTF provided leadership for the development of the plan, proposed specific documents, and worked to obtain faculty buy-in at various steps as the process unfolded. The CRTF conducted a comprehensive literature review and attended curriculum-focused conferences, sessions, and webinars to learn more about current thinking and approaches in curriculum change.

During the exploring phase, the idea of a concept-based curriculum emerged and took hold. First, the CRTF investigated this question: What *IS* a concept-based curriculum? A national expert in conceptual curriculum in nursing (Dr. Jean Giddens) was consulted to conduct a workshop focusing on a concept-based curriculum and concept-based teaching. Members also reviewed documents on integrative learning from the Association of American Colleges and Universities (2000). Forums were held with colleagues in the service sector to inform the CRTF about nursing education issues from the practice perspective. These activities led faculty to conclude that they wanted a concept-based curriculum, but at the same time, a significant question emerged: "How could the college construct a whole curriculum around these ideas?" The next step—*preparing*—allowed faculty to answer that question.

## STEP 3: PREPARING

With the direction set, the work began on the model and the curricular plan. The first step in the *preparing* phase was to identify the crucial concepts. The CRTF identified key concepts from the college's philosophy and framework, as well as the *Essentials of Baccalaureate Education for Professional Practice* (American Association for Colleges of Nursing [AACN], 2008). The CRTF performed a concept sort that led to consensus on a preliminary list of concepts for the curriculum. A curriculum model was designed, and concepts were distributed across the curriculum (Table 3.1).

# TABLE 3.1

## Distribution of Concepts Across Semesters

| Concepts | 266/267 | 265 | 316/317 | 366/367 | 407/507 | 416/417 | 467 |
|---|---|---|---|---|---|---|---|
| **Psychosocial Concepts:** | | | | | | | |
| Adaptation | | | | I | | E | |
| Grief | | | I | E | | E | |
| Health behavior | I,E | | | | | | |
| Interpersonal relationships | | | | I | | | |
| **Physiologic Concepts:** | | | | | | | |
| Pain/comfort | | | I, E | E | | | |
| Thermal regulation | | | | E | | | |
| Metabolic regulation | | | I, E | E | | | |
| Perfusion | | | I, E | E | | | |
| Gas exchange | | | I, E | E | | | |
| Inflammation | | | | I, E | | E | |
| Nutrition | | | | I, E | | E | |
| Elimination | | | | I, E | | E | |
| Skin & tissue integrity | | | I, E | | | | |

(continued)

# TABLE 3.1

## Distribution of Concepts Across Semesters (Continued)

| Concepts | 266/267 | 265 | 316/317 | 366/367 | 407/507 | 416/417 | 467 |
|---|---|---|---|---|---|---|---|
| Mobility | I, E | | E | | | | |
| Immunity | | | | I | | E | |
| Coagulation | | | | I, E | | E | |
| Cognition | I | | | E | | E | E |
| Sensory-perception | I | | | | | E | |
| Anxiety | | | | | | I, E | |
| Fluid & electrolytes | | | I, E | | | | |
| Culture | I, E | | | | | E | E |
| Sexuality | | | | I, E | | E | |
| Spirituality | | | | | | I, E | |
| Vulnerability | | | | | | I, E | E |
| Growth & development | | | | I, E | | | |
| Caring | I, E | | | | | | E |
| Clinical reasoning | | I | E | | | | E |
| Group dynamics | | | | | I, E | E | |

| | | | | | |
|---|---|---|---|---|---|
| Therapeutic communication | | | | I, E | |
| Interpersonal communication | I | | | | |
| Professional communication | I | | E | | E |
| Systems | | I, E | | E | E |
| Quality | I | | | E | E |
| Accountability | I | E | | | E |
| Interprofessional behaviors | I | | I, E | | E |
| Nursing roles | I | E | | E | E |
| Ethics | I | | | E | |
| Legality | | | | I, E | E |
| Health policy | | | | I | E |
| Healthcare economics | I | I | | E | E |
| Standards of practice | I, E | I, E | | | |

LEGEND: I, light or introduction; E, strong emphasis. It is assumed that once the "E" semester occurs, subsequent semesters may be building on the concept.

Additional consultants conducted workshops on campus to provide faculty develop-ment and feedback on the work developed thus far. What concerned faculty the most was the "how to"—how to change the classroom experience, how to develop activities to replace lecture—and worry over "if I don't tell them, they won't understand." The most valuable workshops were those in which the presenter provided broad perspectives and then facilitated the faculty in designing classroom activities and exemplars using their own concepts. This reassured the faculty that they understood and could replicate the process.

## STEP 4: DESIGNING

The *designing* phase moved the faculty's focus to actualizing the curriculum. There was agreement on the big picture points, such as:

1. Foundational skills would be started early and taught in context.
2. Courses would incorporate content across the health continuum.
3. The number of hours of simulation would be increased.
4. Community and mental health content would occur across the curriculum.
5. The program would not be offered during summer semester.

In addition, faculty agreed that there would be no change in the foundational science courses, the length of the program, or the number of credit hours required.

Table 3.2 illustrates the resulting curricular plan. Table 3.3 illustrates the semester components and how the concepts and clinical foci are addressed across the clinical courses.

A faculty retreat was held off campus where templates for syllabi, classroom activities, and lab development were shared. Faculty agreed to post working documents on a com-mon website to prevent duplication as the courses were planned. As the dream turned into a reality, conflicts arose about concept prioritization, movement of individual fac-ulty "pet topics," and responsibility for new topics. During these discussions, it was easy for faculty to return to concern over content rather than concept. Negotiation resulted in a few changes in the concepts and themes, as well as the placement of concepts across the curriculum.

After the retreat, the members of the CRTF shared leadership of small work groups charged with the development of course descriptions, objectives, content, and syllabi. The syllabi were approved by faculty. After this work was completed, the university gov-ernance process began. This process took 1 year, with approval in spring 2011.

## STEP 5: IMPLEMENTING

The *implementing* phase began while awaiting university approval as work continued on the individual courses by teams of faculty who would be involved in implementation of each course. Faculty development continued to be a priority, keeping concept-based teaching as a focus. Faculty were granted release time for course development. Table 3.4 provides an example of how one team integrated concepts across the semester compo-nents of theory, lab, clinical, and simulation.

## TABLE 3.2

## Suggested Pattern of Coursework

| Course | Cr | Course | Cr |
|---|---|---|---|
| Semester 1 | | Semester 2 | |
| BIO 120 General Biology | 4 | CHM 230 Intro to Organic & Biochemistry | 4 |
| CHM 109 Introductory Chemistry | 4 | | |
| PSY 101 Introductory Psychology | 3 | WRT 150 Strategies in Writing | 4 |
| General Education | 3 | BMS 250 Anatomy & Physiology | 4 |
| Total Credits | 14 | General Education | 3 |
| | | Total Credits | 15 |
| Semester 3 | | Semester 4 | |
| BMS 251 Anatomy & Physiology II | 4 | NUR 266 Professional Nursing I | 3 |
| PSY 364 Lifespan Developmental Psychology | 3 | NUR 267 Clinical Nursing I | 5 |
| | | BMS 310 Basic Pathophysiology | 3 |
| BMS 212 Introductory Microbiology | 3 | BMS 305 Clinical Nutrition | 3 |
| BMS 213 Microbiology Lab | 1 | Total Credits | 14 |
| STA 215 Statistics | 3 | | |
| General Education | 3 | | |
| Total Credits | 17 | | |
| Semester 5 | | Semester 6 | |
| NUR 265 Intro Research & Evidence | 3 | NUR 366 Professional Nursing III | 4 |
| NUR 316 Professional Nursing II | 4 | NUR 367 Clinical Nursing III | 6 |
| NUR 317 Clinical Nursing II | 6 | BIO 355 Human Genetics | 3 |
| BMS 311 Pharmacology | 3 | General Education | 3 |
| Total Credits | 16 | Total Credits | 16 |
| Semester 7 | | Semester 8 | |
| IPE 407/507 Interprofessional Communication | 2 | NUR 467 Professional Nursing V | 10 |
| NUR 416 Professional Nursing IV | 4 | General Education | 3 |
| NUR 417 Clinical Nursing IV | 6 | General Education | 3 |
| General Education | 3 | Total Credits | 16 |
| Total Credits | 15 | | |

# TABLE 3.3

## Concepts and Foci Across Clinical Courses

| Semester 4 | Semester 5 | Semester 6 | Semester 7 | Semester 8 |
|---|---|---|---|---|
| **Clinical Focus** | | | | |
| Assessment & Basic Nursing Care | Adult Acute Care & Gerontology | Childbearing & Child Rearing | Severely Mentally Ill & Complex Medical Surgical | Community & Transition into Practice |
| **Clinical Sites** | | | | |
| Long-Term Care/ Subacute | Medical/Surgical | OB/Peds Acute Care | Psych/Mental Health Settings & Acute Care | Communities & Various for Immersion |
| **Mental Health Focus** | | | | |
| Stress, Self-Care, Time Management | Stress, Self-Care, Time Management | Stress, Self-Care, Time Management | Stress, Self-Care, Time Management | Stress, Self-Care, Time Management |
| **Community Focus** | | | | |
| Client in Community— Individual | Client in Community— Context of Family | Community as Client—Aggregate | Community as Client—Community | Community as Client— Vulnerable Population |

## Integration Focus (Simulation)

| Nursing Roles/ Accountability | Fluid/Electrolyte | Perfusion | Grief | Systems |
|---|---|---|---|---|
| • Vital Signs | • Dehydration | • Previa | • End-of-life care | • Mass disaster |
| • Assessment | **Cognition** | • Preeclampsia | **Standards of Practice** | **Nursing Roles** |
| **Safety** | • Delirium | • Post term | • Teamwork | • Multiple patients |
| • Fall Risk Assessment | **Elimination** | • Sickle cell | • Delegation | • Prioritization |
| • Environmental Assessment | • Urinary retention | **Gas Exchange** | **Professional Communication** | • Pediatric, OB, med/ surg |
| **Skin/Tissue** | **Gas Exchange** | • Asthma | • Delegation | **Legality** |
| • Pressure Ulcer Risk Assessment | • Pneumonia | **Metabolic Regulation** | **Nursing Roles** | • Delegation |
| | • COPD | • GDM | • Complex decision-making | |
| | • Post-op | • Hyperemesis | **Vulnerability** | |
| | **Perfusion** | **Grief** | • Human trafficking | |
| | • MI | • Fetal demise | | |
| | • Heart failure | • Abuse (IPV, child) | | |
| | **Metabolic Regulation** | **Safety** | | |
| | • DM ketoacidosis | • Isolation | | |
| | **Safety** | • Medication error | | |
| | • Medication admin. | **Pain/Comfort** | | |
| | **Pain/Comfort** | • Labor | | |
| | • Post-op pain | • Child Appendicitis | | |
| | **Skin/Tissue** | | | |
| | • Burns | | | |
| | **Clinical Reasoning** | | | |
| | • Primary care | | | |

## TABLE 3.4

## Example of How to Integrate Components of Theory, Lab, Clinical, and Simulation Across the Semester

| | 9-Sep | 10-Sep | 11-Sep | 12-Sep | 13-Sep |
|---|---|---|---|---|---|
| 3 | 366: IP Relationships, Growth & Development | 366: Growth & Development | Normal Clinical Hours | Normal Clinical Hours | Normal Clinical Hours |
| | 367 Lab #2 Learning Stations: Developmental Assessment Tools, Prenatal Growth & Development, Gestational Age Assessment, FHR Interpretation | | Clinical Focus: Developmental and Gestational Age Assessments | | |

| | 16-Sep | 17-Sep | 18-Sep | 19-Sep | 20-Sep |
|---|---|---|---|---|---|
| 4 | 366: Pain/Comfort | 366: Nutrition | Peds Groups A, C, E: Normal Clinical Hours | OB Groups A, B, C: Normal Clinical Hours | OB Groups D, E: Normal Clinical Hours |
| | 367 Lab #3 Learning Stations: Pain Scales, Pain Relief in Labor, Positioning in Labor, Breast-feeding, Nutritional Needs for Different Ages, Breast Pumps, NG/GI Tube Feedings | | | Simulations: OB-Peds 15 (fx in pain, varicella) OB-Peds 10 (PPH) | |
| | Clinical Focus: Pain/Comfort, Labor Interventions, Nutritional Needs for Different Ages and Conditions, Breast-feeding | | | | |

| | 23-Sep | 24-Sep | 25-Sep | 26-Sep | 27-Sep |
|---|---|---|---|---|---|
| 5 | Test #1 | 366: Thermoregulation | Normal Clinical Hours | Normal Clinical Hours | Normal Clinical Hours |
| | | No Labs | Clinical Focus: Thermoregulation: Fevers, Newborn Transition | | |
| | 30-Sep | 1-Oct | 2-Oct | 3-Oct | 5-Oct |
| 6 | 366: Gas Exchange | 366: Perfusion | Normal Clinical Hours | Normal Clinical Hours | Normal Clinical Hours |
| | | No Labs | Clinical Focus: Gas Exchange—Effects of Various Conditions, Nursing Interventions, IUGR, Placental Issues | | |
| | 7-Oct | 8-Oct | 9-Oct | 10-Oct | 11-Oct |
| 7 | 366: Perfusion | 366: Coagulation | No Clinical | | |
| | 367 Lab #4 Learning Stations: Cardiac Anomalies, Fetal Circulation, Fetal Heart Monitoring & Interpretation Practice | | Simulations: OB-Peds 19 (sickle cell) OB-Peds 1 (previa) | | |

Of course, there were many issues during the implementation phase, including those related to administration, teaching methodology, and logistics. One administrative issue was related to the loss of the opportunity for teaching during the summer semester, which was possible in the old year-round curriculum. This resulted in a redistribution of faculty workload and a loss of "overload" summer pay. As a result, some faculty chose to teach new courses, such as electives. For some, this opportunity turned out to be a pleasant change of pace.

Other issues arose from the change in pedagogy proposed by the new curriculum design. During the transition from the "old" curriculum to the new curriculum, some faculty found themselves teaching in both curricula during the same semester, causing them to feel further stressed and fractured as they tried to approach teaching in a new way and learning new skills while still needing to finish the old way. However, other faculty responded positively as they reported "trying" concept-based teaching methods in the comfort of the "old" classroom before implementing it in the new curriculum.

Another methodology and a logistical issue was the new integration of simulation. Faculty voted to include 0.5 credits (21 hours) of "integration" in each semester during the clinical course. This represented a change from 0 to 4 hours of simulation per semester to 21 hours of simulation per semester. Faculty agreed during the designing stage that integration would be operationalized by the inclusion of quality, clinical judgment simulations in each clinical course (see Table 3.3). However, during the implementation phase, there was resistance from some faculty about "how to fit it in." It was crucial to have a champion for simulation directly involved in helping each of these course teams develop a plan for implementation of the integration piece of the course. This champion was a faculty member with scholarship in simulation who acted as a consultant for each of the semester planning groups.

## STEP 6: EVALUATING

During the *evaluating* phase, faculty identified student outcomes, student/faculty satisfaction, and course measures. Faculty held debriefings each semester under the auspices of the curriculum committee. Faculty who were teaching their first course in the new curriculum discussed their successes and issues. These discussions were helpful to other faculty as they prepared or revised their own individual courses. Learning from each other stimulated creative thinking, allowed sharing of content, and provided support for both the faculty in the process of implementing a new course and those preparing for a new course. An emerging theme from these sessions was a stated renewed excitement for teaching. Faculty who embraced the idea of concept-based teaching easily followed the lessons from workshops and consulting; however, others had difficulty, and the associate dean provided additional support to those faculty.

Data from faculty evaluations, course evaluations completed by students, and discussions during focus groups were used for formative evaluations. Student reactions to the curriculum changes were both positively and negatively strong. The main issues identified by students were related to pitfalls of first-time offerings, such as a lack of organization, inconsistent communication, and delayed posting of materials in the online system.

Students appreciated the strong emphasis on clinical, simulations, and the variety of teaching methods in the classroom. Additionally, students consistently expressed feelings of being "guinea pigs" in the educational process.

To date, each course in the new curriculum has been implemented a minimum of two times, and faculty are actively engaged in adjusting content and approach. Two cohorts—a traditional generic cohort and a second-degree cohort—graduated in August 2013, having fully experienced the new curriculum. All students took the HESI Exit Exam in their last semester. The new curriculum traditional generic students had the highest mean score compared to scores from previous cohorts. Second-degree students were several points behind but were still at levels near previous cohorts. The highest scores were in community health and professionalism, with values greater than 1,000. Community health had not been a previous strength for the college.

Ninety-five percent of the students who graduated under the new curriculum took the NCLEX-RN© from September 2013 to March 2014, with 91 percent of the candidates passing. The first cohort of the new curriculum scored 4 percent higher than the last cohort of the old curriculum. National pass rates were lower for that period due to changes in the NCLEX-RN passing standard. With the 2014 annual report now available, individual concepts and areas will be assessed.

## SUMMARY

Although the implementation of the new curriculum is considered successful, efforts continue to refine and improve through cycle improvement. Consistency within each course and across the courses (the curriculum) has been identified as an overarching principle. Faculty have found that they must constantly work to keep the content integrated across theory, lab, and clinical experiences within a semester. Whereas in the past faculty were able to silo their work and focus on their own content, the new curriculum requires intense discussion among faculty throughout the undergraduate curriculum. It is important that all faculty have an understanding of how the concepts level across the program. Other areas for attention include the integration of the mental health component across the curriculum and the cohesiveness of the community health component. While mapping the concepts using a different technique, faculty identified a need to reassess placement of the BSN Essentials (AACN, 2008), especially in the early courses.

Last, formal evaluation through employer feedback surveys has not been obtained; however, anecdotal feedback has been positive. The evaluation committee is working on a new survey to obtain this information.

Curriculum change is not an easy process for any nursing program, especially when changing from a content- to a concept-based approach. By awakening faculty interest and commitment, exploring the possibilities, and preparing the college for the change, we were able to design a curriculum that fit the college and prepare our graduates for a successful role in the current and future healthcare system. Implementation of our original plans is complete, but revisions will be ongoing as we continue to respond to the formative and summative measures that we have put in place.

## References

American Association of Colleges of Nursing. (2008). *The essentials of baccalaureate education for professional nursing practice.* Washington, DC: Author.

Association of American Colleges and Universities. (2000). *Greater expectations: A new vision for learning as a nation goes to college.* Available from the Greater Expectations Web site, http://www.greaterexpectations. org/

Benner, P., Stuphen, M., Leonard, V., & Day, L. (2010). *Educating nurses: A call for radical transformation.* San Francisco, CA: Jossey-Bass.

Institute of Medicine. (2000). *To err is human: Building a safer health system.* Washington, DC: National Academies Press.

Institute of Medicine. (2003). *Health professions education: A bridge to quality.* Washington, DC: National Academies Press.

QSEN Institute. (2007). Home Page. Available from QSEN Institute Web site, http://qsen. org

Technology Informatics Guiding Education Reform (TIGER). (2006). The TIGER Initiative. Retrieved June 17, 2015, from http:// www.thetigerinitiative.org/docs/TIGER InitiativeSummaryReport_000.pdf

# 4

# Clinical Experiences in RN-BSN Programs:
## Strategies and Evaluation

**Peggy Hewitt,** MSN, RN

There has been a steady increase in the number of RN-to-BSN programs over the past 10 years (American Association of Colleges of Nursing [AACN], 2013). From 2011 to 2012, programs increased 15.5 percent, and by 2014, there were close to 700 programs, with more than half offering a completely online option (AACN, 2013, 2014). This is encouraging given that 2,906 qualified nurses were turned away from RN-to-BSN programs in 2011 due to a shortage of faculty and resources (AACN, 2012a). This growth in BSN completion programs is also a sign that nursing is moving in the right direction to heed the call from the Institute of Medicine (IOM) for a better-educated nursing workforce (IOM, 2011). Multiple studies have found that better patient outcomes occurred with baccalaureate-prepared nurses (Aiken, Clarke, Cheung, Sloane, & Silber, 2003; Aiken, Friese, Lake, Silber, & Sochalski, 2008; Estabrooks, Midodzi, Cummings, Ricker, & Giovannetti, 2005; Tourangeau et al., 2006; Van den Heede et al., 2009), and the IOM has recommended that 80 percent of RNs be prepared at the baccalaureate level by 2020.

However, as RN-to-BSN programs expand, it is important to ensure that students receive the same quality of education as students graduating from a pre-licensure baccalaureate nursing program. BSN programs not only prepare nurses for a high level of challenge and performance (Hooper, McEwen, & Mancini, 2013) but also provide professional values (Kubesh, Hansen, & Huyser-Eatwell, 2008) and critical thinking (Shin, Jung, Shin, & Kim, 2006). Hendricks et al. (2012) note that BSNs are known for their clinical reasoning and judgment, leadership, health promotion, and application of concepts related to research. The general consensus is that holding these same expectations for RN-to-BSN students is important (AACN, 2012b; McEwen, White, Pullis, & Krawtz, 2012; Rodriguez, McNiesh, Goyal, & Aspen, 2013). RN-to-BSN programs must maintain high standards to graduate professional nurses with these attributes. If not, RN-to-BSN programs could risk the reputation of "dumbing down" degree requirements, leaving the BSN degree portrayed as meaningless (McEwen, Pullis, White, & Krawtz, 2013). This chapter reviews the literature of strategies and evaluation methods used to enhance nursing knowledge through practice experiences in RN-to-BSN programs.

# REVIEW OF THE LITERATURE

An initial CINAHL search of "RN to BSN" and "Post RN" resulted in 20 peer-reviewed research articles from the years 2011 through 2014. The search was narrowed using "RN to BSN" and "Clinical Evaluation"; however, that search did not yield any peer-reviewed research during that same time. Adding the word "education" to "RN to BSN" also did not yield any results. "RN to BSN" and "Practice Experience" resulted in one study using reflective practice, whereas "RN to BSN Program" and "Clinical" resulted in three studies: one focusing on community health, one on comfort with genetics in RN-to-BSN students, and one related to clinical competence of students.

The search was expanded to include the years 2010 through 2014 using the search terms "RN-BSN" and "Evaluation." This resulted in 14 studies that included topics such as cultural competence, online programs, critical thinking, emergency preparedness, and new graduate skills. A national research study looking at RN-to-BSN programs was the only study that examined programs since the IOM's call for more baccalaureate-prepared nurses (McEwen et al., 2012).

Recognizing the growing number of RN-to-BSN programs, the AACN created a task force to clarify expectations for clinical practice experiences for these students in 2012 (AACN, 2012b). Although RN-to-BSN programs in accredited institutions must meet the AACN's *Essentials of Baccalaureate Education for Professional Nursing Practice* (AACN, 2008), the *Essentials* do not differentiate between pre-licensure BSNs and RN-to-BSNs. Therefore, the task force published *White Paper: Expectations for Practice Experiences in the RN to Baccalaureate Curriculum,* recommending experiences to transition the associate's degree nurse to the role of the baccalaureate nurse (AACN, 2012b). The paper offers general guidance for the clinical component in completion programs; however, there is little in the literature on effective clinical strategies and methods of evaluation for transitioning associate's degree nurses to the role of the baccalaureate-prepared nurse.

Nurses in completion programs bring knowledge and experience to the classroom and the practicum. The literature repeatedly notes that RN-to-BSN students are a distinct population; they have their own learning needs (Allen & Armstrong, 2013; Asselin, 2011; Conner & Thielemann, 2013; Ezeonwu, Berkowitz, & Vlasses, 2013; Hendricks et al., 2012) and require a separate set of outcome measures (Hooper et al., 2013; McEwen et al., 2012, 2013; Robertson, Canary, Orr, Herberg, & Rutledge, 2010). This is important to consider when planning practice experiences for these students.

RN-to-BSN students have already achieved the basic skills required for entry-level practice. Allen and Armstrong (2013) compare the clinical learning needs of these students to those of graduate students in terms of focusing on learning outcomes instead of time on task. Allowing students to design their own clinical learning plan with assistance from faculty provides an opportunity for students to address their areas of interest and possible future professional plans (Allen & Armstrong, 2013). Students can take advantage of this experience to explore unknown environments and broaden their view of nursing.

Few studies have examined clinical experiences in RN-to-BSN programs. Further, there is little evidence of consistency in programs (Hendricks et al., 2012; McEwen et al., 2012, 2013). In fact, a national survey of RN-to-BSN programs found large variations in RN-to-BSN completion programs (McEwen et al., 2012, 2013). These variations included not only curriculum content but also clinical evaluation and clinical requirements. At the time of the survey, approximately 16 percent of the completion programs had no clinical component. Also of note, there was considerable variation in required clinical hours, areas of clinical focus, and evaluation methods.

Required hours varied from 15 to 180 for community nursing and 16 to 270 for leadership, with the average number being just under 80 hours (McEwen et al., 2012). The most common areas of clinical focus were community and public health, with leadership/management and role transitions the second most common areas. Some schools incorporated a clinical experience into courses such as health assessment, critical care, health promotion, or gerontology (McEwen et al., 2012). Papers, projects, and clinical logs were the most common form of clinical evaluation, with preceptor input and self-evaluation (or peer evaluation) frequently used.

In one school, RN-to-BSN students in a leadership course used reflection to gain perspective on the relationship of course content to practice (Asselin, 2011). This course did not have a practicum; however, through reflective journals, online assignments and posts, 1-minute papers, and audio-taped interviews, students reflected on current practice in relation to course content and on strategies to facilitate change using knowledge gained from the course. Students in the course stated that the reflection strategies allowed them to link key concepts learned in the course to their own area of practice.

## CLINICAL EVALUATION AND STRATEGIES FOR RN-TO-BSN STUDENTS

Clinical evaluation for licensed nurses is very different from evaluation of pre-licensure students. The most common method of clinical evaluation for RN-to-BSN students is a paper or project (McEwen et al., 2012). Clinical logs and preceptor input are also ranked high as methods used to evaluate students. Self- and peer evaluation are common methods of clinical evaluation. Surprisingly, 46 percent of the respondents were "frequently" or "always" evaluated through instructor observation (McEwen et al., 2012). It is not clear whether these were "observations" of student presentations or observations of students' interactions in a clinical setting.

The most common evaluation strategy for RN-to-BSN students is the use of self-reflection through journaling or discussion board posts. These strategies for evaluating practice experiences have been shown to be successful in enhancing RN-to-BSN students' learning (Asselin, 2011; Ezeonwu et al., 2013; Northrup-Snyder, Van Son, & McDaniel, 2011). Ezeonwu et al. (2013) noted that the current model of nursing education emphasizes acute care skills and is not adequate for today's healthcare needs. Using a blend of online and face-to-face learning with community integration, Ezeonwu et al. (2013) implemented a community practice experience for RN-to-BSN students. Students posted reflections online and responded to classmates' posts by analyzing their observations, activities, and readings. This blended approach allowed the RNs to work with a population with whom they seldom interacted. The approach also enhanced the integration of critical thinking and research skills, provided opportunities to use leadership skills and planning and evaluation skills, increased cultural awareness and sensitivity, and improved communication skills. In addition, students with acute care backgrounds learned to focus on the health of the population rather than the care of an individual (Ezeonwu, 2013).

Northrup-Snyder et al. (2011) used online discussions to reflect on clinical experiences of RN-to-BSN students in a community course. Two themes emerged:

1. Awareness of the community and the context of public and community health nursing roles; and

2. Understanding the transitions of patients from home to the hospital and back to the home.

Using reflection strategies led to a greater understanding of community and public health by RN-to-BSN students (Northrup-Snyder et al., 2011).

One study reviewed integrating evidence-based practice (EBP) into an RN-to-BSN practicum to improve EBP efficacy and decrease barriers to research utilization (Oh et al., 2010). The practicum period followed a two-credit course on nursing research methodology. Students applied the knowledge by defining a patient problem in their assigned clinical practice setting, selecting the best nursing intervention based on the level of evidence, and considering how the evidence could be applicable to their patient. Student conferences were held to discuss progress during this precepted experience. The clinical semester ended with presentations to faculty members (Oh et al., 2010). A pre-test/post-test revealed a statistically significant increase in scores on EBP efficacy and a significant decrease in barriers to research utilization (Oh et al., 2010).

Students in a completely online RN-to-BSN program submitted projects or other artifacts from practice experiences to the school's faculty evaluators (Jones-Schenk, 2014). A standardized rubric was used for grading to ensure that competencies were met. Projects were graded by a faculty member serving in the role of evaluator, whereas other faculty members were either course mentors or student mentors (Jones-Schenk, 2014). Faculty roles in this program were disaggregated to allow members to serve where they were most suited to support best faculty practices.

## DISCUSSION

Clinical education, or practice experience, is a critical component of nursing education. Such experience allows nurses the opportunities to integrate newly acquired knowledge and skills into practice. Pre-licensure nursing education integrates theory and practice in clinical experiences that teach students to "think like a nurse" (Benner, Sutphen, Leonard, & Day, 2010, p. 12). It is through these experiences that students learn to "put it all together," applying concepts learned in the didactic setting in the clinical arena with real patients under the supervision of licensed nurses. Not only do pre-licensure nursing programs have clinical components, but graduate nursing programs also have required practice experiences and expectations (AACN, 2012c). Regardless of the level of education, nursing is a practice discipline that reflects a higher level of clinical practice with each increase in the level of education.

Clinical education is at the heart of preparing nurses with the knowledge, skills, and attitudes needed to improve quality and safety in health care. This is the overall thrust of the Quality and Safety Education for Nurses Institute (QSEN Institute, 2014). Knowledge, skills, and attitudes, which are as important as the nursing process itself, are enhanced during practice experiences and are used to promote the professionalism of the nurse.

The most common clinical practice strategy used in RN-to-BSN programs is that of reflection, which provides an opportunity to think through situations. These situations are often emotionally charged. The process allows students to make sense of their actions and reactions, and consider how they might handle a similar situation in the future. Gaining such awareness can lead to improved patient outcomes and a reduction in errors (Sherwood & Horton-Deutsch, 2012). RN-to-BSN students' knowledge and appreciation for community, public health, and leadership increase when reflection strategies are combined with online discussions and assignments. Altmann (2012) noted that nurses who returned to school to continue formal education had more positive attitudes. A more positive attitude, combined with greater awareness of nursing practice discovered through reflection, will lead to a better-educated and more knowledgeable nursing workforce. However, there is clearly a need for more research on clinical experiences for RN-to-BSN students.

These students, who are already licensed nurses, may have learning needs that not only meet the *Essentials* but also may even surpass those criteria. Having already demonstrated basic competence for practice as an entry-level RN, experienced RNs returning for a BSN are ready to move beyond the immediate concerns of entry-level practice. Studies exploring other areas of nursing, such as systems thinking and processes, gerontology, informatics, and policy, as well as more EBP, are needed to discover their fit into the RN-to-BSN curriculum.

## RECOMMENDATIONS

The gap in the literature on practice experiences for nurses in BSN completion programs points to the need to not only identify clinical learning strategies for this population of students but also identify practice experiences best suited for nurses with varying years of experience. Addressing the learning styles and needs of RN-to-BSN students with varied experience has always been a challenge. A recent study by McEwen et al. (2013) found that more than 46 percent of RN-to-BSN program directors were noticing an increase in the number of students with less experience. These students are younger and have a different level of preparation than students in the past (McEwen et al., 2013). Alongside these new nurses, there may be an older RN with years of experience seeking a BSN due to pressure from the employer. It has been noted that experienced RNs returning to school under duress often present with more challenging attitudes (Altmann, 2012). Although it is encouraging that nurses are enrolling in completion programs earlier in their career, schools of nursing must be prepared to meet the differing needs of the changing population of students.

Evaluation of practice experiences is another area that would benefit from further research. Clinical evaluation traditionally has been difficult for nurse educators, especially when a student is not performing well (Lewallen & DeBrew, 2012). This raises many questions concerning the evaluation of clinical practice experiences in RN-to-BSN programs. What methods are being used to determine where students are in the learning process? What are effective methods for clinical evaluation, particularly if a student is not doing well? How many practice hours do RN-to-BSN students need to successfully transition into the BSN role? Should practice hours be competency based and individualized at the student level? How much value do instructors place on student practice experiences? What would it look like for RN-to-BSN students to have practicum experiences in their place of employment?

Ensuring that practice experiences are individualized to "grow nurses," meet the *Essentials* and other learning outcomes, and offer the level of education offered to prelicensure BSN students is vital to the advancement of nursing. This is true whether the nurse is a new graduate or a nurse with many years of experience. Nurse educators must stay abreast of the ever-changing population of RN-to-BSN students. Clinical learning strategies for RN-to-BSN students must continually be evaluated to ensure that students' needs are met. Quality education cannot be disregarded for the purpose of moving students through the system. It must be evident that a nurse previously practicing at the associate's degree level is now practicing as a baccalaureate-prepared nurse. Most importantly, evaluation of completion programs must be an ongoing process. Dialogues regarding expectations and standards for completion programs need to be open and frank. As associate's degree nurses are encouraged to pursue a higher level of education, it is only fair they receive a high level of excellence in their educational program in return. Providing RN-to-BSN students with exceptional educational experiences not only will contribute to improved healthcare delivery but also will raise the bar for the profession of nursing.

## ACKNOWLEDGMENT

The author gratefully acknowledges the editorial assistance of Ms. Elizabeth Tornquist, MA, FAAN, and the assistance of Mrs. Dawn Wyrick with this manuscript.

## *References*

Aiken, L. H., Clarke, S. P., Cheung, R. B., Sloane, D. M., & Silber, J. H. (2003). Educational levels of hospital nurses and surgical patient mortality. *Journal of the American Medical Association, 290*(12), 1617–1623.

Aiken, L. H., Friese, C. R., Lake, E. T., Silber, J. H., & Sochalski, J. (2008). Hospital nurse practice environments and outcomes for surgical oncology patients. *Health Services Research, 43*(4), 1145–1161.

Allen, P. E., & Armstrong, M. L. (2013). RN-BSN curricula: Designed for transition, not repetition. *Journal of Professional Nursing, 29*(6), e37–e42.

Altmann, T. K. (2012). Nurses' attitudes toward continuing formal education: A comparison by level of education and geography. *Nursing Education Perspectives, 33*(2), 80–84.

American Association of Colleges of Nursing. (2008). *The essentials of baccalaureate education for professional nursing practice.*

Retrieved June 17, 2015, from http://www.aacn.nche.edu/education-resources/BaccEssentials08.pdf

American Association of Colleges of Nursing. (2012a). *2012 annual report. Leadership, collaboration, innovation: Advancing higher education in nursing.* Retrieved June 17, 2015, from http://www.aacn.nche.edu/aacn-publications/annual-reports/AnnualReport12.pdf

American Association of Colleges of Nursing. (2012b). *White paper: Expectations for practice experiences in the RN to baccalaureate curriculum.* Retrieved June 17, 2015, from http://www.aacn.nche.edu/aacn-publications/white-papers/RN-BSN-White-Paper.pdf

American Association of Colleges of Nursing. (2012c). *Criteria for evaluation of nurse practitioner programs.* Retrieved June 17, 2015, from http://www.aacn.nche.edu/education-resources/evalcriteria2012.pdf

American Association of Colleges of Nursing. (2013). *2013 annual report. Moving the conversation forward: Advancing higher education in nursing.* Retrieved from http://www.aacn.nche.edu/aacn-publications/annual-reports/AnnualReport13.pdf

American Association of Colleges of Nursing. (2014). *Fact sheet: Degree completion programs for registered nurses: RN to master's degree and RN to baccalaureate programs.* Retrieved January 25, 2015, from http://www.aacn.nche.edu/media-relations/DegreeComp.pdf

Asselin, M. E. (2011). Using reflection strategies to link course knowledge to clinical practice: The RN-to-BSN student experience. *Journal of Nursing Education, 50*(3), 125–133.

Benner, P., Sutphen, M., Leonard, V., & Day, L. (2010). *Educating nurses: A call for radical transformation.* San Francisco, CA: Jossey-Bass.

Conner, N. E., & Thielemann, P. A. (2013). RN-BSN completion programs: Equipping nurses for the future. *Nursing Outlook, 61*(6), 458–465.

Estabrooks, C. A., Midodzi, W. K., Cummings, G. G., Ricker, K. L., & Giovannetti, P. (2005). The impact of hospital nursing characteristics on 30-day mortality. *Nursing Research, 54*(2), 74–84.

Ezeonwu, M., Berkowitz, B., & Vlasses, F. (2013). Using an academic-community partnership model and blended learning to advance community health nursing pedagogy. *Public Health Nursing, 31*(3), 272–280.

Hendricks, S. M., Phillips, J. M., Narwold, L., Laux, M., Rouse, S., Dulemba, L., et al. (2012). Creating tomorrow's leaders and innovators through an RN-to-bachelor of science in nursing consortium curricular model. *Journal of Professional Nursing, 28*(3), 163–169.

Hooper, J. L., McEwen, M., & Mancini, M. E. (2013). A regulatory challenge: Creating a metric for quality RN-to-BSN programs. *Journal of Nursing Regulation, 4*(2), 34–38.

Institute of Medicine. (2011). *The future of nursing: Leading change, advancing health.* Washington, DC: National Academies Press.

Jones-Schenk, J. (2014). Nursing education at Western Governors University: A modern, disruptive approach. *Journal of Professional Nursing, 30*(2), 168–174.

Kubesh, S., Hansen, G., & Huyser-Eatwell, V. (2008). Professional values: The case for RN-BSN completion education. *Journal of Continuing Education in Nursing, 39*(8), 375–384.

Lewallen, L. P., & DeBrew, J. K. (2012). Successful and unsuccessful clinical nursing students. *Journal of Nursing Education, 51*(7), 389–395.

McEwen, M., Pullis, B. R., White, M. J., & Krawtz, S. (2013). Eighty percent by 2020: The present and future of RN-to-BSN education. *Journal of Nursing Education, 52*(10), 549–557.

McEwen, M., White, M. J., Pullis, B. R., & Krawtz, S. (2012). National survey of RN-to-BSN programs. *Journal of Nursing Education, 51*(7), 373–380.

Northrup-Snyder, K., Van Son, C. R., & McDaniel, C. (2011). Thinking beyond "the wheelchair to the car:" RN-to-BSN student understanding of community health and public health nursing. *Journal of Nursing Education, 50*(4), 226–229.

Oh, E. G., Kim, S., Kim, S. S., Kim, S., Cho, Y., Yoo, J.-S., et al. (2010). Integrating evidence-based practice into RN-to-BSN clinical nursing education. *Journal of Nursing Education, 48*(7), 387–392.

QSEN Institute. (2014). Project Overview. Retrieved June 17, 2015, from http://qsen.org/about-qsen/project-overview/

Robertson, S., Canary, C. W., Orr, M., Herberg, P., & Rutledge, D. N. (2010). Factors related to progression and graduation rates for RN-to-bachelor of science in nursing programs: Searching for realistic benchmarks. *Journal of Professional Nursing, 26*(2), 99–107.

Rodriguez, L., McNiesh, S., Goyal, D., & Aspen, L. (2013). Methods of evaluating an accelerated associate degree registered nurse to baccalaureate degree continuation program. *Journal of Professional Nursing, 29*(5), 302–308.

Sherwood, G. D., & Horton-Deutsch, S. (2012). *Reflective practice: Transforming education *and improving outcomes.* Indianapolis, IN: Sigma Theta Tau International.

Shin, K., Jung, D. Y., Shin, S., & Kim, M. S. (2006). Critical thinking dispositions and skills of senior nursing students in associate, baccalaureate, and RN-to-BSN programs. *Journal of Nursing Education, 45*(6), 233–237.

Tourangeau, A. E., Doran, D. M., Hall, L. M., Pallas, L. O., Pringle, D., Tu, J. V., et al. (2006). Impact of hospital nursing care on 30-day mortality for acute medical patients. *Journal of Advanced Nursing, 57*(1), 32–44.

Van den Heede, K., Lesaffre, E., Diya, L., Vleugels, A., Clarke, S. P., Aiken, L. H., et al. (2009). The relationship between inpatient cardiac surgery mortality and nurse numbers and educational level: Analysis of administrative data. *International Journal of Nursing Studies, 46*(6), 796–803.

# 5

# Integrating Mental Health Nursing in a Baccalaureate Curriculum

**Caralise W. Hunt,** PhD, RN

**William Stuart Pope,** DNP, RN, DMin

**Jenny B. Schuessler,** PhD, RN

Mental health is an integral component of overall health (World Health Organization [WHO], 2014). It is estimated that 43.7 million Americans age 18 years and older suffer from mental illness. This represents approximately 19 percent of the U.S. population (National Institute of Mental Health, 2012). A recent WHO survey of 28 countries found mental illness prevalence rates between 18 and 36 percent, with the United States having one of the highest rates (Kessler et al., 2009).

Mental and physical health are inextricably linked. A person's mental health affects the ability to maintain physical health. People with severe mental illness are more likely to have comorbid physical conditions including cardiovascular disease, type 2 diabetes, pulmonary disease, and liver disease (Leue et al., 2010). Physical health problems impact treatment of mental health problems, and mental illness affects participation in healthy behaviors. To address this problem, the U.S. Department of Health and Human Services (HHS) established a Healthy People 2020 goal to increase the proportion of primary care facilities that provide mental health treatment (HHS, 2011).

In the acute care setting, patients with mental health conditions are frequently admitted to medical units for treatment of nonpsychiatric conditions. Care of these patients may be suboptimal due to underutilization of mental health treatment guidelines, inadequate education and training of staff, and stereotyping and stigma from staff (MacNeela, Scott, Treacy, Hyde, & O'Mahony, 2012). Additionally, the attitudes of nurses working on general hospital units toward patients with mental illness have been described as negative (Zolnierek, 2009).

In all healthcare contexts, due to complex needs of persons with mental health issues, nurses play a vital role in the holistic care of patients. Although mental health care has been recognized as an essential aspect of health care (Institute of Medicine [IOM], 2011), there is a lack of adequate training for nurses who provide this care (WHO, 2007). Lack of educational preparation may leave nurses feeling apprehensive and vulnerable when caring for patients with mental health conditions (Buckley, 2010). Koch and Whittaker (1985) suggested that teaching psychological concepts in a separate course makes it difficult to apply these concepts to clinical practice. Effective education, on the other hand, has been found to positively impact student nurses' attitudes about mental health nursing (Ferrario, Freeman, Nellett, & Scheel, 2008; Happell & Gaskin, 2012; Heise, Johnsen, Himes, & Wing, 2012).

The American Psychiatric Nurses Association (APNA, 2008) recommends that students be exposed to essential psychiatric/mental health nursing concepts across the entire baccalaureate curriculum. Mental health content and learning outcomes vary across the lifespan and settings, and they are best taught across the curriculum rather than in one course or semester (APNA, 2008). Increased exposure to mental health concepts and patients living with mental illness may decrease nurses' negative responses to these patients (Zolnierek, 2009). This chapter describes the revision and integration of mental health curricular content across one baccalaureate nursing curriculum.

## BACKGROUND AND SIGNIFICANCE

Nursing students are exposed to mental health patients in a variety of practice settings. These patients require psychological support, and students are expected to provide that support. Appropriate educational preparation regarding mental health conditions is essential for undergraduate nursing students so that they are ready to care for these patients in various practice areas (Buckley, 2010). However, mental health nursing traditionally has been taught in blocked semester theory and clinical psychiatric nursing courses, with mental health rarely mentioned in other courses. This delivery method limits the ability of students to develop and apply knowledge and skills in therapeutic communication, therapeutic relationships, and clinical reasoning in the care of patients with mental illness in settings other than those formally designated for psychiatric care.

Nurses can play a key role in implementing effective care to patients with mental illness in both psychiatric and nonpsychiatric settings. To be effective, students must comprehend the relevance of the application of mental health knowledge and skills to care for these patients. Furthermore, the integration of mental health nursing content throughout nursing education and experience may promote nurses' self-confidence in caring for patients with mental illness and, in turn, improve their attitudes about these patients (Zolnierek, 2009). Integrated mental health content should continue to be taught by specialists who have mental health knowledge and expertise (Happell & McAllister, 2014).

In the current healthcare environment, a better understanding and a more integrated view of mental health care is needed to enhance healthcare delivery (Roberts, Robinson, Stewart, & Smith, 2009). Expanding mental health content in nursing curricula, ensuring that adequate mental health theoretical content is integrated within all nursing courses, and providing clinical placements across a variety of settings throughout the curriculum provide support for and may improve competency in mental health nursing for students who encounter patients living with mental illness (Warelow & Edward, 2009).

## DEVELOPMENT AND GOALS OF THE MENTAL HEALTH CURRICULUM

In response to the societal need for more comprehensive mental health care, faculty at one baccalaureate nursing program developed an innovative approach to mental health nursing. This innovation integrated mental health concepts throughout the curriculum and was part of an overall curriculum revision. The goal of integrating mental health nursing was to increase exposure to mental health concepts and expand opportunities to practice mental health skills. Integration of mental health throughout the curriculum encourages and facilitates the practice of holistic care by students.

The conceptual framework of the curriculum was based on aspects from a variety of nursing theories and emphasized awareness of and respect for individual patient perceptions and needs (Erickson, Tomlin, & Swain, 1983). Important foundations of the conceptual framework included developing therapeutic relationships, promoting health, preventing disease, and applying evidence-based knowledge in a culturally sensitive, compassionate, and patient-centered manner. These curricular foundational concepts were the basis for integration of mental health content across the curriculum.

In undertaking curriculum redesign, faculty also attended to the limitations of the formerly nonintegrated curriculum. Baccalaureate students in this nursing program had voiced concerns about their unfamiliarity with mental illness during their first mental health clinical experience at a community mental health facility during the second semester of the nursing program. They also had indicated through qualitative comments and course evaluation feedback that they were unsure how to begin conversations and uncertain about what to discuss with patients; consequently, they felt that the mental health clinical experiences were not beneficial.

Faculty members also observed interactions between nursing students and mental health patients and found that students either avoided engaging patients or discussed nontherapeutic social topics with patients. The communication scores of students on standardized tests were below benchmark as well. After evaluation of student course evaluations, standardized tests, and clinical observations, faculty determined that the problem was not with the clinical experience but instead with students' preparation for and approach to the experience.

Philosophically, faculty believed that good communication skills were the foundation from which a nurse with strong mental health nursing skills would emerge. They espoused the guidelines of the APNA (2008), which state that psychosocial content is the core for all areas of nursing and that content such as therapeutic communication should be introduced early in the nursing curriculum. Faculty frequently observed students having difficulty communicating with peers, faculty members, patients, and other healthcare professionals. The overwhelming majority of students in this school of nursing were Millennials, born between 1982 and 2000. Therefore, generational factors and inexperience may have contributed to the communication issues. The faculty attended to all of these issues and goals, with due consideration of relevant literature.

## LITERATURE REVIEW

The Millennial Generation's preferred method of communication is through electronic media (Beard, Schwieger, & Surendran, 2008). This generation of students was raised with email, texting, and Facebook®. These students are capable of increased efficiency due to technology but find it difficult to work without it (Marston, 2010). Because of limited face-to-face interactions, Millennials may interpret nonverbal communication poorly, and their verbal communication may suffer as a result (Beard et al., 2008). Deas (2011) states that 90 percent of the cues people receive in conversation are nonverbal. This leads to problems with verbal communication, and specifically therapeutic communication.

As many as 1 in 10 young people struggle to form relationships because their speech, language, and communication difficulties go unrecognized (Larson & McKinley, 2003).

Students often express anxiety about interacting with patients living with mental illness (Kameg, Howard, Clochesy, Mitchell, & Suresky, 2010). Students may be unfamiliar with mental illness and may have been exposed to social stigmas associated with mental illness, resulting in the presence of fear toward these patients (Brown, 2008).

The issue of whether to implement integrated or nonintegrated mental health curriculum content has been discussed in the literature, but the emphasis is on integrated clinical experiences rather than integrated theoretical content. No studies or reviews related to integrated versus nonintegrated theoretical mental health content were identified in the literature review.

Due to the lack of resources for mental health care, the WHO (2008) recommends integrating mental health into primary care to ensure access to mental health care. Mental health care can be integrated into primary care clinical experiences. Faculty at one school of nursing developed a clinical rotation experience to provide mental and physical health care for patients in a primary care setting (Roberts et al., 2009). Family nurse practitioner and mental health nurse practitioner students worked with a team consisting of a family nurse practitioner, psychiatrist, and family practice physician to provide integrated mental health care for patients in a primary care clinic. This qualitative study revealed strengthened learning experiences and improved nursing skills in providing mental health care. Integration of mental health care into primary care settings is also being incorporated into doctor of nursing practice curricula (Burgermeister, Kwasky, & Groh, 2012).

One article described an integrated clinical experience for undergraduate students (Faught, Gray, DiMeglio, Meadows, & Menzies, 2013). Baccalaureate nursing students completed a clinical rotation on a medical or surgical unit with the goals of providing holistic, integrated mental and physical health care; increasing awareness of and improving perceptions regarding mental illness; and expanding understanding of the importance of the nurse-patient relationship. Qualitative evaluations of the clinical experience revealed several students realizations that regardless of a patient's medical diagnosis or unit assignment, mental health is an important part of the patient's care. Other students found it difficult to talk to patients about their mental health when they were on a medical or surgical unit and staff nurses were not addressing mental health issues. With all of this experiential and formal knowledge, the faculty proceeded to design the integration of mental health content throughout their baccalaureate nursing curriculum.

## BUILDING COMMUNICATION SKILLS IN THE FIRST AND SECOND SEMESTERS

In the integrated curriculum, communication principles are the focus in the first two semesters to address deficits in communication skills and promote development of therapeutic relationships. The first nursing course provides an overview of therapeutic communication techniques because of their importance and impact on patient care in all settings. Students participate in theoretical and practical learning experiences to develop therapeutic communication skills.

A didactic unit on therapeutic communication is included in the fundamentals nursing course. This course also includes labs that provide opportunities for students to practice communication with simulated patients, peers, and other healthcare providers. Students interact with patients during a mock hospital simulation that occurs before they begin clinical experiences. Faculty observe these interactions and discuss skills performance and therapeutic communication techniques with students following the simulation. In another lab, students pair to practice interviewing for a health history. Finally, students have the opportunity to practice interprofessional and situation, background, assessment, and recommendation (SBAR) communication during clinical laboratory practices. Once all laboratories have been completed, students have the opportunity to practice therapeutic communication with patients in acute care and community settings.

The second semester clinical course is a major building block integrating mental health into the curriculum. The clinical course combines medical-surgical and psychiatric nursing concepts. Faculty work with staff at the outpatient mental health clinic to develop a list of practical life skills topics for students to discuss with patients. Students learn about commonly occurring mental health disorders, including anxiety, situational crisis, depression, and delirium. The role of the mental health nurse in the community is taught in this course. Additionally, instruction is provided about caring for acutely ill patients with preexisting mental health conditions in medical-surgical situations.

In this course classroom, simulation laboratory and traditional clinical experiences are interwoven in a manner that enhances application of concepts learned in previous courses and critical thinking. For example, each student has the opportunity to work in both an outpatient mental health clinic with a mental health nurse and in a prison setting with a mental health counselor. In these settings, students participate in groups and also work individually with clients. Therapeutic communication is reinforced by the healthcare professionals working with the students. Students provide patients with a 15- to 20-minute presentation on a topic, such as personal hygiene, tips for visiting the doctor, and weather safety. Patients then ask questions or comment on the topic. These presentations provide a means for students to lead conversations with patients, with the goal of therapeutic discussions about a patient's mental health. Additionally, these clinical experiences offer opportunities to teach people living with mental health conditions about health promotion and disease prevention.

An especially innovative technique used to teach mental health concepts in the curriculum is simulation. Simulation provides an avenue for teaching mental health concepts, including therapeutic communication (Brown, 2008). Simulation experiences have been successful in increasing self-confidence and self-efficacy for communication with mental health patients (Kameg et al., 2010). Videos and scenarios that simulate psychiatric patients and situations may dispel student anxieties before they encounter actual patient care (Brown, 2008).

The first of three simulations focusing on mental health occurs in this second semester course. In this simulation scenario, students encounter a chronically ill child's anxious mother, who is dealing with multiple life stressors. The students learn to use therapeutic communication to decrease the mother's anxiety and resolve a situational crisis.

Faculty added a communication lab to the second semester to improve mental health clinical experiences. The lab involves a simulated situation in which students must therapeutically communicate with a standardized patient. Students first view a video of a therapeutic interaction between a nurse and a mental health patient. Following the video, students role-play a communication scenario with a standardized patient. At the conclusion of the scenario, students complete an interpersonal record that provides an opportunity to reflect on their communication and identify strengths and weaknesses. These learning experiences meet Millennials' learning needs by including active participation and immediate feedback desired by this generation (Marston, 2010).

## PULLING IT ALL TOGETHER IN THE THIRD AND FOURTH SEMESTERS

The third semester of the integrated curriculum focuses on mental health principles applied to diverse and vulnerable populations. This community-focused class discusses socioeconomically disadvantaged populations, such as the homeless, migrants, and pregnant teens. Societal issues including abuse, violence, and drug and alcohol addiction are explored as both a cause and result of mental illness. The impact of these societal issues on the ability to access mental health care is studied. Clinical experiences include postnatal teen mother visits and prison health. Students lead health fairs and outreach projects in which they teach vulnerable populations such as migrant workers, well elderly, and at-risk teens. This course has achieved two unexpected outcomes:

1. Students learn that mental health issues are encountered wherever one goes in the community.

2. There is often a lack of mental health resources in the United States.

Students internalize these realities to a degree that could never be accomplished in a classroom setting.

The decision to integrate mental health across the curriculum was made with the commitment that mental health would be enhanced, not minimized. The goal was for mental health nursing to be truly "integrated" rather than "disintegrated." Therefore, it was important that the curriculum include a course with content and clinical experience typically taught in a mental health course. In this curriculum, that course is in the fourth semester. As part of a clinical course focusing on chronic and complex conditions, mental health conditions that require inpatient hospitalization are included. Concepts in this course include schizophrenia, bipolar disorder, major depressive disorder, suicide, eating disorders, and personality disorders. This course also includes a long-term care component with end of life, palliative care, elder abuse, and primary dementia. Students engage in 48 hours of structured clinical experience in an inpatient psychiatric facility and 24 hours in a skilled nursing home environment. During clinical time, students are exposed to severe mental illness. Students are required to participate in inpatient groups and perform extensive mental health assessments. Students identify a mental condition and explore best practices in caring for this condition, reinforcing evidence-based practice.

Placing an inpatient mental health experience in the fourth semester rather than earlier in the curriculum has had a synergistic effect. This experience gives students the opportunity to practice the mental health concepts and competencies they learned throughout the curriculum within an intensive setting. Previously, the inpatient mental health rotation was in the third semester. Affording students an extra semester of experience has improved students' ability to adapt to the unfamiliar settings; locked units; and patients experiencing acute, severe mental illness. This course placement allowed them greater opportunity to apply evidence-based knowledge in a culturally sensitive, compassionate, patient-centered manner.

Two simulation experiences in this course provide consistent exposure to mental health concepts in a safe, controlled environment. The first simulation experience exposes students to an asthmatic patient with schizophrenia. The purpose of this scenario is to emphasize that wherever nursing is practiced, persons with mental illness will be encountered. Students work through this complex situation to address the physiological problems that are compounded by the mental illness and the mental illness that is complicated by the physiological problems. The second simulation scenario in this course is an end-of-life situation in which cultural differences require cultural humility and sensitivity to achieve therapeutic communication and end-of-life care. These simulations ensure that all senior students have equal opportunity to work through multifaceted complex situations in a safe, supportive environment. A structured debriefing process promotes self-reflection and learning.

## EVALUATION

The purpose of integrating mental health concepts across the curriculum was to increase exposure to mental health concepts and expand opportunities to practice mental health skills. The impetus for integration was not to improve examination or standardized test scores, but to provide a more comprehensive view of mental health nursing concepts. However, we did explore learning outcomes by examining standardized test results. Students in the five-semester nursing curriculum take standardized tests that measure mental health concepts in four of the five semesters and take one standardized psychiatric test during the fourth semester. Following administration of each standardized test, faculty examine test results for areas of student strength and weakness in mental health concepts including communication, abuse, psychoses, depression, anxiety, and grief and loss. Mean scores in these areas are compared to benchmark, and institutional results are compared to national results.

Standardized psychiatric test scores using Health Education Systems Incorporated (HESI) exams prior to integration were at or above benchmark. Following integration, standardized test scores remained consistent with test scores prior to implementing the integrated curriculum, suggesting that the approach did not undermine learning outcomes. In fact, several areas in standardized test scores have indicated gains in learning outcomes. Performance on psychiatric and mental health concepts within nonpsychiatric standardized tests has increased since the mental health content was integrated into the curriculum. Specifically, psychiatric and mental health concepts within the Pharmacology standardized test, which is administered in the second semester, increased significantly from 938 to 1,157 ($p < .05$). This finding suggests that earlier exposure to mental health concepts is beneficial for nursing students. With the intense focus on communication in the first and second semesters, standardized test scores for communication have exceeded benchmarks, ranging from 913 to 1,012. Faculty comments on students' clinical evaluations reflect an improvement in therapeutic communication skills.

## CONCLUSION

When mental health nursing content was integrated throughout one baccalaureate curriculum rather than taught in one specific course, students came to realize early in the curriculum that holistically caring for a patient includes being aware of the patient's mental state. One student commented that "the clinical setting doesn't matter, I am always dealing with mental health issues." This curriculum revision started with a focus on basic communication skills and built on that foundation to include acute, chronic, and complex psychiatric concepts. Teaching strategies varied and included simulation, skills laboratories, analysis of videos, and focused assignments related to clinical practice opportunities. Qualitative and quantitative evaluation has indicated that integrating mental health nursing theory and practice throughout a baccalaureate curriculum effectively promotes attention to mental health throughout all aspects of nursing care.

## References

American Psychiatric Nurses Association & International Society of Psychiatric Mental Health Nurses. (2008). *Essentials of psychiatric mental health nursing in the BSN curriculum.* Retrieved June 18, 2015, from http://www.apna.org/files/public/revmay08finalCurricular_Guidelines_for_Undergraduate_Education_in_Psychiatric_Mental_Health_Nursing.pdf

Beard, D., Schwieger, D., & Surendran, K. (2008). Preparing the millennial generation for the work place: How can academia help? In *Proceedings of the 2008 ACM SIGMIS CPR Conference on Computer Personnel Doctoral Consortium and Research* (pp. 102–105). New York, NY: ACM.

Brown, J. F. (2008). Applications of simulation technology in psychiatric mental health nursing education. *Journal of Psychiatric and Mental Health Nursing, 15*(8), 638–644.

Buckley, S. (2010). Caring for those with mental health conditions on a children's ward. *British Journal of Nursing, 19*(19), 1226–1230.

Burgermeister, D., Kwasky, A., & Groh, C. (2012). Promoting mental health concepts in a doctor of nursing practice curriculum: An integrated and global approach. *Nurse Education in Practice, 12*(3), 148–152.

Deas, R. (2011). Technology is the devil in disguise. *Liberty Champion.* Retrieved June 18, 2015, from http://www.liberty.edu/champion/2011/11/technology-is-the-devil-in-disguise/

Erickson, H. C., Tomlin, E., & Swain, M. A. (1983). *Modeling and role-modeling: A theory and paradigm for nursing.* Upper Saddle River, NJ: Prentice Hall.

Faught, D. D., Gray, P., DiMeglio, C., Meadows, S., & Menzies, V. (2013). Creating an integrated psychiatric-mental health nursing clinical experience. *Nurse Educator, 38*(3), 122–125.

Ferrario, C. G., Freeman, F. J., Nellett, G., & Scheel, J. (2008). Changing nursing students' attitudes about aging: An argument for the successful aging paradigm. *Educational Gerontology, 34*(1), 51–66.

Happell, B., & Gaskin, C. J. (2012). The attitudes of undergraduate nursing students towards mental health nursing: A systematic review. *Journal of Clinical Nursing, 22*(1–2), 148–158.

Happell, B., & McAllister, M. (2014). Implementing a major stream in mental health nursing: Barriers to effectiveness. *International Journal of Mental Health Nursing, 23*(5), 435–441.

Heise, B. A., Johnsen, V., Himes, D., & Wing, D. (2012). Developing positive attitudes toward geriatric nursing among millennials and generation Xers. *Nursing Education Perspectives, 33*(3), 156–161.

Institute of Medicine. (2011). *Essential health benefits: Balancing coverage and cost.*

Retrieved June 18, 2015, from http://books. nap.edu/openbook.php?record_id=13234

Kameg, K., Howard, V. M., Clochesy, J., Mitchell, A. M., & Suresky, J. M. (2010). The impact of high fidelity human simulation on self-efficacy of communication skills. *Issues in Mental Health Nursing, 31*(5), 315–323.

Kessler, R. C., Aguilar-Gaxiola, S., Alonso, J., Chatterji, S., Lee, S., Ormel, J. et al. (2009). The global burden of mental disorders: An update from the WHO World Mental Health (WMH) Surveys. *Epidemiologiae psichiatria sociale, 18*(1), 23–33. Available from http://www.ncbi.nlm.nih.gov/pmc/articles/PMC3039289/

Koch, H., & Whittaker, K. (1985). Teaching psychology to psychiatric nurses: Revision and implications. *Nurse Education Today, 5*(3), 109–113.

Larson, V. L., & McKinley, N. L. (2003). Service delivery options for secondary students with language disorders. *Seminars in Speech and Language, 24*(3), 181–198.

Leue, C., Driessen, G., Strik, J. J., Drukker, M., Stockbrugger, R. W., Kuijpers, P. M., et al. (2010). Managing complex patients on a medical psychiatric unit: An observational study of university hospital costs associate with medical service use, length of stay, and psychiatric intervention. *Journal of Psychosomatic Research, 68*(3), 295–302.

MacNeela, P., Scott, P. A., Treacy, M., Hyde, A., & O'Mahony, R. (2012). A risk to himself: Attitudes toward psychiatric and choice of psychosocial strategies among nurses in medical-surgical units. *Research in Nursing & Health, 35*(2), 200–213.

Marston, C. (2010). *How to train millennials.* Mobile, AL: Generational Insight.

National Institute of Mental Health. (2012). *Prevalence: Any mental illness among adults.* Retrieved June 18, 2015, from http://www.nimh.nih.gov/health/statistics/prevalence/any-mental-illness-ami-among-adults.shtml

Roberts, K. T., Robinson, K. M., Stewart, C., & Smith, F. (2009). An integrated mental health clinical rotation. *Journal of Nursing Education, 48*(8), 454–459.

U.S. Department of Health and Human Services, Healthy People 2020. (2011). *Mental health and mental disorders.* Retrieved June 18, 2015, from http://www.healthypeople.gov/2020/topicsobjectives2020/overview.aspx?topicid=28

Warelow, P., & Edward, K. L. (2009). Australian nursing curricula and mental health recruitment. *International Journal of Nursing Practice, 15*(4), 250–256.

World Health Organization. (2007). *Atlas: Nurses in mental health: 2007.* Geneva, Switzerland: Author.

World Health Organization. (2008). *Integrating mental health into primary care: A global perspective.* Geneva, Switzerland: Author.

World Health Organization. (2014). *Mental health: Strengthening our response.* Fact sheet N220. Retrieved June 18, 2015, from http://www.who.int/mediacentre/factsheets/fs220/en/

Zolnierek, C. D. (2009). Non-psychiatric hospitalization of people with mental illness: Systematic review. *Journal of Advanced Nursing, 65*(8), 1570–1583.

# 6

# Ethical Grand Rounds:
## Teaching Ethics at the Point of Care

**Norah M. M. Airth-Kindree,** DNP, MSN, RN
**Lee-Ellen C. Kirkhorn,** PhD, RN

The baccalaureate nursing program at the University of Wisconsin, Eau Claire, offers an educational innovation called *Ethical Grand Rounds* (EGR) as a teaching strategy to enhance ethical decision-making. Nursing students participate in EGR-flexible ethical laboratories, where they take stands on ethical dilemmas, arguing for—or against— an ethical principle. This process provides the opportunity to move past *normative ethics,* an ideal ethical stance in accord with ethical conduct codes, to *applied ethics,* what professional nurses would do in actual clinical practice, given the constraints that exist in contemporary care settings. EGR serves as a vehicle to translate "what ought to be" into "what is."

Although nursing is among the nation's most trusted professions (Gallup, Inc., 2013), there has been considerable professional commentary on a national and international level regarding the causes and effects of what has been termed the *compassion deficit.* It has been suggested that nurses need to reestablish kindness, caring, and compassion as core professional values (Blakemore, 2011; McHale, 2012; Peate, 2012). Ethical shortcomings in care may begin in the classroom and extend into clinical practice.

Some suggest that nurses who overlook ethical principles are those who attended school years ago, when there were no ethical questions on the licensure exam and ethics was not a required part of the nursing curriculum. However, a review of the literature revealed a dearth of evidence to support such a claim. One study (Ham, 2004) suggested that practicing nurses with more than 6 months of experience are more likely to conform rather than question current practices. Findings indicate that new graduates initially act based on individual moral codes, only gradually succumbing to environmental pressures for conformity.

Although ethics education is threaded throughout the typical nursing program and includes the *Code of Ethics for Nurses* of the American Nurses Association (2001) and philosophy courses in nursing education, nurses are confronted with real-life barriers that make ethical practice difficult (De Casterlé, Izumi, Godfrey, & Denhaerynck, 2008). Such barriers include pressure to conform, too few resources (human and financial), and little administrative support. Tschudin (2013) reports that nursing students are likely to say, "First let me learn all that I need to pass my exams, and then I will think about ethics if there is any time left" (p. 123).

# RATIONALE FOR THE INNOVATION

Most nursing theory courses help students become socialized into the profession, giving them confidence in the psychomotor skills of practice. Approaches to real-world ethical choices have not had the same level of curricular attention (Buchman & Porock, 2005). Students are not universally instructed in how to proceed in circumstances where an ethical course of action is ambiguous or when faced with troubling ethical dilemmas.

Practicing nurses confront dilemmas concerning the allocation of scarce resources (e.g., organ donation), budget constraints and poor staffing ratios, horizontal workplace violence (e.g., the emotional battering of a colleague), and telling the truth about medication errors. In our experience as nurse educators, most nursing students, and many practicing nurses, say that their socialization into the practice of professional nursing neither prepared them to apply ethics at the point of care nor provided opportunities to examine decisions. Baldwin (2010) notes a "disconnect between nursing education (where students are taught the ideal) and the real world of nursing (where compromises about what should be done and what can be done occur daily)" (p. 5).

Nursing students often respond to sterile objective classroom hypotheticals by insisting, "I would never do that. Period. End of statement." Nursing students may be embarrassed to appear uncaring or considered unethical before their peers when contemplating an unacceptable ethical option—even for a classroom hypothetical situation.

The classroom ethical "front" that nursing students present is often short lived. Once students descend from the purity of the ivory tower into the real world, where they can no longer "afford" the virtues of academic purity, the hypothetical situations of the classroom or virtual environment may fall by the wayside. The descent might not be nearly as precipitous had nurse educators offered instruction in ethics at the point of care coupled with nursing theory courses. EGR facilitates the development of students' critical thinking in resolving ethical dilemmas by the proper application of ethical principles, not simply by appeal to emotion.

# ETHICAL GRAND ROUNDS

Our program is a traditional baccalaureate program in a public university in the Midwest. We incorporated a two-part EGR into a sophomore Foundations of Care clinical experience in a long-term care setting for 56 students enrolled in their first clinical experience.

## Part 1

For the first part of the EGR, participants, primarily female, were divided into clinical sections of eight students per clinical instructor. Following clinical each week, instructors and students met in a postconference at the clinical site to discuss specific topics—ethical dilemmas derived from the instructors' actual clinical practice experiences. These included end-of-life decision-making, understaffing issues, covering for a co-worker, and HIPAA. During this conference, normative ethical principles, as described in the *Code of Ethics for Nurses* (ANA, 2001) were corporately reviewed.

## BOX 6.1

### Ethical Grand Rounds Part 1: Example of an Ethical Dilemma for Nursing Student Discussion

Mrs. Jones, a patient with Alzheimer's disease (AD), had great difficulty eating without choking. She was hospitalized for a choking episode and then transferred to a long-term care facility. Her family notified the staff that she must have assistance when eating.

Several days later, a meal was brought to the patient's room. Your friend, Margie, who is a certified nursing assistant (and fellow classmate in your BSN program), told you that she was working that day and was assisting another patient when she found Mrs. Jones slumped over in a chair.

Upon investigation, the cause of death was found to be asphyxiation from food in her throat. Your classmate tells you that a wrongful death suit is going be brought against the long-term care facility for breaches of the standard of care. She is very fearful of losing her job.

Your classmate claims that she was not informed about the importance of assisting the patient when eating, and she begs you never to tell anyone that no one provided assistance to the patient.

Complicating matters is the fact that you know your classmate really needs employment, and you believe that she is telling the truth when she says she was not told about the patient's condition. You also believe that there were breaches of the standard of care.

You are absolutely convinced that your classmate will be fired if she steps forward and tells her side of the story to nursing administration.

What will you do? Why?

For each of two clinical sections, there were four groups and four topic exemplars (see one example in Box 6.1). Students discussed ethical dilemmas by using normative principles as adversaries (e.g., paternalism vs. autonomy/fidelity vs. beneficence). They sat across from each other at a table and debated the merits of the ethical principle they had chosen to defend for each case study.

A limitation of this part of the EGR is that case studies derived from faculty experience are not representative of the full domain of clinical dilemmas in practice. Evolving issues, such as data sharing, computerized documentation systems, deontology, and utilitarianism, were not addressed; only ethical principles of autonomy, beneficence, fidelity, nonmaleficence, paternalism, and veracity were reviewed with students. The narrowly focused demographic composition of the nursing student sample also limited the debate.

## Part 2

To reinforce the application of didactic content, a postclinical discussion topic was assigned for asynchronous completion within a course management system. Within clinical groups, students were required to address diverse themes and respond to colleagues in a substantive manner. The instructor served as facilitator and provided a summation of the discussions.

Faculty discussion leaders asked that students describe an ethical situation personally encountered in clinical that week, applying an ethical principle. In addition, students were prompted to incorporate the ABCDE ethical decision-making model, derived from their classroom text (Black, 2014), and describe how they came to the decision they ultimately acted upon. This model, which offers a template for helping students resolve ethical dilemmas at the point of care, has the following five steps:

1. Clarify the ethical dilemma
2. Gather additional data
3. Identify options
4. Make a decision/act
5. Evaluate

Students had much to share during this assignment and readily identified ethical dilemmas that they had encountered. Some students revealed that it was easier to make an ethical decision when they felt passionate about an ethical dilemma. One student reported that knowing ethical principles was the factor that helped to determine her decision; by promoting beneficence, she fulfilled the nursing role of patient advocate. Discussions overall indicated that students felt comfortable taking action on ethical dilemmas according to such principles as caring, respect, and patient safety.

Other ethical dilemmas were not as easy for students to address. Indeed, some nursing students felt powerless in their role, not wanting to upset staff or clients. Consequently, some ethical issues noted (e.g., inappropriate talk by staff while providing personal care) were overlooked and not attended to at all. Certainly the relative lack of experience and expertise among neophyte nursing students were limiting factors for the application of ethical principles discussed in the EGR.

## IMPLICATIONS FOR STUDENTS AND NURSING PRACTICE

The feeling of powerlessness or moral distress is not unique to students. As Varcoe et al. (2004) observed in their study of ethical practice in nursing, nurses were "often torn between doing the right thing and not jeopardizing their potential to do good in the future" (p. 323). As patient advocates, all healthcare workers, whether in the student or professional role, should have ethical conviction and confidence to advocate at the point of care.

A theoretical and clinical ethical underpinning in foundational nursing courses supports ethical practice. As De Casterlé et al. (2008) point out, "It is of utmost importance that nurses are capable to practice following higher ethical reasoning to bring the greatest benefit to patients" (p. 547). Scholarly educational research is needed to determine the impact of teaching ethics at the point of care using EGR. Possible research questions include the following examples: How do graduates of EGR approach ethical problems once they become practicing nurses? What additional clinical and didactic opportunities are needed to enhance ethical practice? How confident do EGR graduates feel when handling ethical problems?

Given responses from nursing students, it appears that even when knowledge of ethical principles is present at the point of care, acting on ethical principles is not a consistent finding. Perhaps nursing clinical role models—more effectively than most—can show neophyte practitioners how they themselves dealt with ethical quandaries early in life. How did successful practicing nurses navigate ethical minefields early on in their clinical experience? Did they falter? If so, how quickly did they recover? And if they faced the need to navigate those same fields once again, what would they do differently?

## CONCLUDING THOUGHTS

Our experience suggests that students' conscious and deliberate focus to justify an ethical course of action required considerable critical thinking. It became clear that ethical dilemmas had no easy solutions and, at times, could not be resolved. Just as De Casterlé et al. (2008) noted among practicing nurses, there are varying levels of difficulty when following through with ethical decisions under challenging circumstances.

From our perspectives, ethical dilemmas are commonplace, complex, and require critical thinking skills that are honed through practice, practice, and more practice. We offer EGR as one innovative strategy for nursing education and suggest that even more clinical evidence is needed to determine its long-term effectiveness with students.

### References

American Nurses Association. (2001). *Code of ethics for nurses: Provisions.* Retrieved June 18, 2015, from www.nursingworld.org/codeofethics

Baldwin, K. M. (2010). Moral distress and ethical decision-making [Editorial]. *Nursing made incredibly easy.* Retrieved June 18, 2015, from http://journals.lww.com/nursingmadeincrediblyeasy/toc/2010/10000

Black, B. P. (2014). Ethics: Basic concepts for nursing practice. In B. P. Black (Ed.), *Professional nursing: Concepts and challenges* (7th ed., pp. 88–112). St. Louis, MO: Saunders.

Blakemore, S. (2011). New health commission to tackle poor care issues. *Nursing Older People, 23*(7), 6–7.

Buchman, D., & Porock, D. (2005). A response to C. Varcoe, G. Doane, B. Pauly, P. Rodney, J. L. Storch, K. Mahony, G. McPherson, H. Brown, & R. Starzomski (2004), "Ethical practice in nursing: Working the in-betweens." Journal of Advanced Nursing 45(3), 316–325. *Journal of Advanced Nursing, 51*(6), 658–659.

De Casterlé, B., Izumi, S., Godfrey, N. S., & Denhaerynck, K. (2008). Nurses' responses to ethical dilemmas in nursing practice: Meta-analysis. *Journal of Advanced Nursing, 63*(6), 540–549.

Gallup, Inc. (2013). *Honesty/ethics in professions.* Retrieved June 18, 2015, from www.gallup.com/poll/1654/Honesty-Ethics-Professions.aspx

Ham, K. (2004). Principled thinking: A comparison of nursing students and experienced nurses. *Journal of Continuing Education in Nursing, 35*(2), 66–73.

McHale, J. V. (2012). The ageing population: Is it time for an international convention of rights? *British Journal of Nursing, 21*(6), 372–373.

Peate, I. (2012). Kindness, caring and compassion [Editorial]. *Australian Nursing Journal, 19*(7), 16.

Tschudin, V. (2013). Two decades of nursing ethics: Some thoughts on the changes. *Nursing Ethics, 20*(2), 123–125.

Varcoe, C., Doane, G., Pauly, B., Rodney, P., Storch, J. L., Mahony, K., et al. (2004). Ethical practice in nursing: Working the in-betweens. *Journal of Advanced Nursing, 45*(3), 316–325.

# 7

# Teaching-Learning Strategies in a Concept-Based Curriculum

**Carmen V. Harrison,** MSN, RNC
**Sharon K. Pittard,** MSN, RNC

In nursing education, there are concerns about content overload (Hardin & Richardson, 2012) and curricular designs that focus on disease processes. According to Giddens and Brady (2007), a medical model focus is inappropriate for the nursing profession. One solution that streamlines the delivery of instructional material and emulates nursing practice is a concept-based curriculum (Hardin & Richardson).

Concept-based curricula facilitate learning through the recognition and analysis of connections between concepts (Giddens & Brady, 2007). Essential concepts are identified and defined for stages of the learning process. As students progress through the curriculum, they apply conceptual information from previous courses to their new courses and clinical experiences (Giddens & Brady; Giddens, Wright, & Gray, 2012; Hardin & Richardson, 2012).

## ACTIVE TEACHING-LEARNING STRATEGIES

Although considered effective in the past, lecture-based teaching (Popkess & McDaniel, 2011) is now thought to be antiquated and ineffective for today's nursing student (Fairman & Okoye, 2011). Lecture-based teaching is inadequate for preparing nursing students with the skill sets necessary to provide care for patients with multifaceted healthcare conditions (Fairman & Okoye). Active teaching-learning strategies are found to be superior to lecture-based teaching in preparing nurse graduates to transition from the student to the practitioner role (Fairman & Okoye).

Active learning has been defined as the generation of knowledge among students who are engrossed and involved in the learning process (Greer, Pokorny, Clay, Brown, & Steele, 2010). Guiding this process is a faculty member who serves as a facilitator in teaching or disseminating information to students (Greer et al.). A concept-based curriculum supports the execution of active teaching-learning strategies that focus on a particular concept or similar group of concepts.

Students' ability to comprehend and synthesize information is augmented through the use of active teaching-learning strategies in a concept-based curriculum (Giddens & Brady, 2007). Concept maps, in which students illustrate an analysis of associations among various concepts (Hardin & Richardson, 2012), are an example of a popular active teaching-learning strategy used in concept-based curricula.

## CRITICAL THINKING

Healthcare-related errors continue to be an alarming concern (Institute of Medicine [IOM], 2001, 2006). Effective critical thinking by novice nurses decreases mishaps within healthcare environments (Fero, Witsberger, Wesmiller, Zullo, & Hoffman, 2009). Critical thinking has been defined as the ability to use logic to analyze information in clinical decision-making, identifying the rationale for these decisions, and recognizing when to implement alternative options (Fero et al.).

Nurse educators can prepare new graduates to make clinical decisions founded on sound critical thinking through the use of educational practices aimed at developing this cognitive ability (Fairman & Okoye, 2011). The relationship between a concept-based curriculum, active teaching-learning strategies, and critical thinking has been established (Giddens & Brady, 2007; Hardin & Richardson, 2012).

## IMPLEMENTING ACTIVE TEACHING-LEARNING STRATEGIES

Prior to adopting a concept-based curriculum at the project site, a nurse faculty task force was charged with conducting a review of the literature and critiquing the articles to determine appropriateness for inclusion/exclusion. The literature search primarily used the Cumulative Index to Nursing and Allied Health Literature (CINAHL), the Education Resources Information Center (ERIC), and PubMed by incorporating the subject terms "concept-based curriculum," "nursing curriculum," "nursing education," and "education, nursing associate" for the years 2000 through 2009.

Members of the task force attended continuing education seminars focused on concept-based curricula. Findings and recommendations identified by members of the task force on the process for transitioning to a concept-based curriculum and the utilization of active teaching-learning strategies were routinely shared with all nursing faculty. Thus, curriculum revision decisions were made by consensus.

Consultation with a content expert took place prior to the placement of concepts into the curriculum. This ensured continuity and prevented the inadvertent loss of vital educational content. Each selected concept within the revised curriculum related to the patient, the nursing profession, and the healthcare system.

Faculty collaborated to construct learning focus guides for every class within each course. These learning focus guides provided a definition for the concept and listed the related exemplar(s), learning outcomes, learning resources, active teaching-learning activities, and methods for evaluating student learning. A similar process for implementing a concept-based curriculum was described by Giddens and Brady (2007).

Sections of the revised curriculum required a decrease in specialized content, such as obstetrical nursing, in both the classroom and clinical settings. Although this approach is commonly associated with a concept-based curriculum (Giddens & Brady, 2007), the faculty members assigned to this course were challenged by the need to deliver condensed and relevant information with innovative and active teaching-learning strategies. Whereas previous knowledge of many of the concepts in the curriculum, such as infection and perfusion, was easily transferred from course to course, the concept of reproduction was only covered in this specific course, creating a greater dilemma for faculty.

## REPRODUCTION IN THE REVISED CURRICULUM

In the revised curriculum, the concept of reproduction was presented in three individual classes and associated with exemplars for antepartum, intrapartum, postpartum, prematurity, and newborn care. Learning outcomes created for each class directed the active teaching-learning activities and were utilized to assess student learning. Each class required students to complete an assignment prior to class so that class time could be spent on theoretical application of the content and discussion.

An unfolding case study utilized as an active teaching-learning strategy followed a patient through the antepartum, intrapartum, and postpartum periods. The teaching-learning strategies involved clinical scenarios and related questions. Upon completion of the unfolding case study, students discussed the answers.

Other active teaching-learning strategies allowed students to listen to simulated fetal heart tones and to view uterine contraction patterns via a computerized program. High-fidelity manikins were used for clinical scenarios where students actively participated in newborn care and care of an antepartum, intrapartum, and postpartum patient. With another active teaching-learning strategy, students used pelvic and fundal models to identify and describe normal and abnormal fundal assessments of the antepartum and postpartum patient.

## COURSE EVALUATIONS

Course evaluation data provided positive comments by students. Students reported that the use of active teaching-learning strategies helped them develop knowledge of the reproduction concept and transfer this information from the classroom to the clinical setting. Assessment summaries of student learning and faculty statements regarding student classroom and clinical performance were favorable as well.

Although this curriculum revision remains in the infancy stage of operation at this project site, plans are in place to perform rigorous research to explore the outcome of active teaching-learning strategies in a concept-based curriculum. Given that the literature has suggested that active teaching-learning strategies in a concept-based curriculum promote the development of students' critical thinking ability (Giddens & Brady, 2007; Hardin & Richardson, 2012), evaluation of critical thinking scores will be used to determine the effect of this curriculum revision.

---

## References

Fairman, J. A., & Okoye, S. M. (2011). Nursing for the future, from the past: Two reports on nursing from the Institute of Medicine. *Journal of Nursing Education, 50*(6), 305–311.

Fero, L. J., Witsberger, C. M., Wesmiller, S. W., Zullo, T. G., & Hoffman, L. A. (2009). Critical thinking ability of new graduate and experienced nurses. *Journal of Advanced Nursing, 65*(1), 139–148.

Giddens, J. F., & Brady, D. P. (2007). Rescuing nursing education from content saturation: The case for a concept-based curriculum. *Journal of Nursing Education, 46*(2), 65–69.

Giddens, J. F., Wright, M., & Gray, I. (2012). Selecting concepts for a concept-based curriculum: Application of a benchmark approach. *Journal of Nursing Education, 51*(9), 511–515.

Greer, A., Pokorny, M., Clay, M. C., Brown, S., & Steele, L. L. (2010). Learner-centered characteristics of nurse educators. *International Journal of Nursing Education Scholarship, 7*(1), 6–15.

Hardin, P. K., & Richardson, S. J. (2012). Teaching the concept curricula: Theory and method. *Journal of Nursing Education, 51*(3), 155–159.

Institute of Medicine. (2001). *Crossing the quality chasm: A new health system for the 21st century.* Washington, DC: National Academies Press.

Institute of Medicine. (2006). *Preventing medication errors.* Washington, DC: National Academies Press.

Popkess, A. M., & McDaniel, A. (2011). Are nursing students engaged in learning? A secondary analysis of data from the National Survey of Student Engagement. *Nursing Education Perspectives, 32*(2), 89–94.

# Students Collaborating to Improve Learning

**Kathleen DeLeskey,** DNP, RN, CNE, FJBI
**Gretchen Rosoff,** MEd, RN

Nursing education is driven by numerous identified local and national initiates that are rapidly changing the direction of nursing practice. The Institute of Medicine (IOM) and the Robert Wood Johnson Foundation released the 2010 report *The Future of Nursing: Leading Change, Advancing Health,* which described the need for a new structure that provides nurses with expanded education and skills to meet the current and future healthcare needs (IOM, 2010). Among other elements, the mandate petitions for an increase in the number of baccalaureate and higher educationally prepared nurses and assurance that lifelong learning will be an inherent part of the profession.

The Quality and Safety Education for Nursing (QSEN) Institute, initially created in 2005, introduced six criteria for nurses to ensure competent practice and patient safety in health care. The criteria are patient-centered care, teamwork and collaboration, evidence-based practice, quality improvement, safety, and informatics (QSEN Institute, 2014a).

In August 2010, the Massachusetts Department of Higher Education and Massachusetts Organization of Nurse Executives along, with other important stakeholders from state and national commissions, created the Massachusetts Nurse of the Future (NOF) committee. This committee produced the report *Building the Framework for the Future of Nursing Education and Practice* (Invitational Working Session, 2006). The intent of the Massachusetts NOF was to inform future nursing practice and curricula to encompass those same QSEN competencies (Sroczynski, Gravlin, Seymore Route, Hoffart, & Creelman, 2011).

With broad educational mandates and preparation of nurses shifting to meet current healthcare needs, nurse educators are seeking new and progressive ways to teach to replace the constantly growing list of skills and competencies. Nurses of the future must be ready to respond and continue to learn in a fluid healthcare environment.

There is a significant body of literature demonstrating that nursing students are often highly stressed in the clinical setting (Moscaritolo, 2009; Christiansen & Bell, 2012; Jimenez, Navia-Osorio, & Diaz, 2010). This supports faculty experiences of students expressing feelings of being "overwhelmed" and "stressed out" when beginning clinical practice. Moreover, medical literature describes that extreme anxiety among newly qualified physicians can escalate to panic, rendering them unable to make any treatment decisions (Tallentire,

Smith, Skinner, & Cameron, 2011). Clearly, anxiety and stress have an impact on student performance in the clinical setting. Given that the obligation of nurse educators is to prepare nurses who are able to respond and continue to learn in a fluid healthcare environment, addressing anxiety becomes an essential part of preparing nurses of the future.

Although human patient simulators are used to prepare students for the clinical practice environment, our students continue to complain that they prefer to "take care of a real person before I have to go do it on an actual patient." In an effort to facilitate NOF and QSEN recommendations while considering student input, faculty met to brainstorm and develop a learning strategy that would meet the learning needs of students and prepare them to be nurses of the future. This lab experience was designed to allay clinical anxiety by allowing new nursing students the opportunity to practice skills in a safe, nonthreatening environment prior to beginning patient care in the hospital setting.

Laboratory objectives for the new students were to:

1. Take part in a therapeutic communication experience in a safe environment.
2. Practice physical assessment skills with an experienced peer.
3. Use critical thinking to evaluate the needs of a patient and family in a team meeting.

The senior objectives were to:

1. Establish a mentoring role with a novice nursing student.
2. Assist a novice student to experience a professional nurse-patient relationship.
3. Demonstrate professional nursing skills for a new nursing student.

Once the objectives were established, we identified clinical scenarios that would allow students to attain their goals. After the senior students became familiar with their roles, they conducted the laboratory sessions while faculty served only as available resources for assistance.

## FORMAT OF THE EXPERIENCE

The lab consisted of four sections that occurred simultaneously. Each senior student was assigned a role for the duration of the lab. Novice students rotated through the four sections to elicit the maximum learning experience.

The first section consisted of a few seniors who individually spent time with two or three novices while sharing a video provided on the QSEN website called *The Lewis Blackman Story* (QSEN Institute, 2014b). This true story depicts the outcome of a medical error that cost the life of a child. The small groups watched the video together and discussed the issues surrounding the experience, with seniors acting as guides. The encounter was intended to guide critical thinking and teamwork while focusing on patient safety.

The second section served the purpose of allowing novice students to practice therapeutic communication with patients. Senior students were given their assigned role a few days prior to the lab. Each had a simple medical diagnosis with a secondary issue that was unknown to the novice. The issues included such things as a husband who just told his hospitalized wife that he wants a divorce, and hospitalization following a motor vehicle accident in which the best friend who was a passenger was killed. The new students were instructed to visit with the patient and have a therapeutic discussion with the patient. The conversations were left entirely up to the student role-playing the patient and the novice student. Following the discussion, the seniors reinforced good communication skills and helped to guide novice skills.

The third section provided patients (seniors) in a bed, and the novice students were charged with completing a head-to-toe assessment and a set of vital signs. The "patients" demonstrated the signs and symptoms of the assigned disease while students completed an assessment. Following the assessment, seniors spent time pointing out the positive aspects of the assessment and guiding the novices in ways to improve the assessment and make it easier to complete. The focus here was collaboration and evidence-based practice.

The final section was a collaborative team meeting. Faculty created a short (4-minute) video depicting a nurse caring for a 59-year-old patient with metastatic bone disease. The patient is in a great deal of pain and wishes to die but tells the nurse that her daughter will not let her go. The team views the video together, then proceeds to the "meeting." The seniors are assigned roles as the primary care physician, social worker, distraught daughter, respiratory therapist, and hospital chaplain. They are given advance notice of their roles. The novice students arrive for the meeting and are assigned roles at the door. They are the nurses and nursing assistants caring for the patient. Each team member acts out his or her role based on the information from the video. An ethical dilemma is presented, and it is up to the professional team to arrive at a consensus about further treatment for the patient. This section was totally focused on teamwork and collaboration.

## DISCUSSION

We have completed the three semesters using this approach to learning. After each session, we made small changes based on student feedback. Students stated that the sessions were a positive learning experience. Seniors remarked that they "did not realize I knew so much" and "it was so much fun to help the new students." In fact, *all* seniors described feeling positive and having a "great time" during the experience. Seven of them wrote, "Wish we had this when we were novices!"

Novice students wrote statements such as "they taught me so much" and "it helped a lot to do vital signs and a head-to-toe with the seniors helping." Many wrote that "the seniors were so helpful and they know so much." One particularly articulate student wrote that "the teamwork session was very vivid and gave me a sense of the reality of the patients and their family members involved in decisions related to their health."

## CONCLUSION

In addition to providing our novice students with a safe and nonthreatening clinical lab experience, we sought to demonstrate to our graduating seniors the critical role of a nurturing mentor in the profession. The faculty intend for these students to serve as mentors and nurturers as part of their professional roles. Additionally, the level of competency and empathy of new graduates may help to decrease the number of medical errors each year that are reportedly contributing to more than 200,000 American deaths each year (Andel, Davidow, Hallander, & Morendo, 2012).

# References

Andel, C., Davidow, S., Hallander, M., & Morendo, D. (2012). The economics of health care quality and medical errors. *Journal of Health Care Finance, 31*(9), 39–50.

Christiansen, A., & Bell, A. (2012). Peer learning partnerships: Exploring the experience of pre-registration nursing students. *Journal of Clinical Nursing, 19*(5–6), 803–810.

Institute of Medicine. (2010). *A summary of the October 2009 forum on the future of nursing: Acute care.* Washington, DC: National Academies Press.

Invitational Working Session. (2006). *Creativity and connections: Building the framework for the future of nursing education and practice.* Retrieved June 18, 2015, from http://www.mass.edu/currentinit/documents/NursingCreativityAndConnections.pdf

Jimenez, C., Navia-Osorio, M., & Diaz, C. (2010). Stress and health in novice and experienced nursing students. *Journal of Advanced Nursing, 66*(2), 442–455.

Moscaritolo, L. (2009). Interventional strategies to decrease nursing student anxiety in the clinical learning environment. *Journal of Nursing Education, 48*(1), 17–23.

QSEN Institute. (2014a). *Pre-licensure KSAS.* Retrieved June 18, 2015, from http://qsen.org/competencies/pre-licensure-ksas/

QSEN Institute. (2014b). *The Lewis Blackman story.* Retrieved June 18, 2015, from http://qsen.org/faculty-resources/videos/the-lewis-blackman-story/

Sroczynski, N., Gravlin, G., Seymore Route, P., Hoffart, N., & Creelman, P. (2011). *Creativity and connections: The future of nursing education practice: The Massachusetts Initiative.* Retrieved June 18, 2015, from http://www.mass.edu/currentinit/documents/nursing/nofarticle.pdf

Tallentire, V., Smith, S., Skinner, J., & Cameron, H. (2011). Understanding the behaviour of newly qualified doctors in acute care contexts. *Medical Education, 45*(10), 995–1005.

# 9

# Teaching Graduate Students Evidence-Based Practice

**Alyce S. Ashcraft,** PhD, RN, CNE, ANEF
**Carol Boswell,** EdD, RN, CNE, ANEF
**Yondell Masten,** PhD, WHNP-BC, RNC-OB
**Mary Madeline Rogge,** PhD, RN, FNP-BC
**Kellie Bruce,** PhD, RN, FNP-BC
**Steve Branham,** PhD, RN, ACNP-BC, FNP-BC, FAANP
**Joanna Guenther,** PhD, RN, FNP-BC, CNE

Clinician integration of skill, expertise, and judgment with clinically relevant research evidence must consider the accuracy and precision of physical assessment and diagnostic techniques, along with safety, efficacy, and comparative costs of preventive or therapeutic interventions, as well as client preferences. The American Association of Colleges of Nursing (AACN, 2011) and the National Organization of Nurse Practitioner Faculties (NONPF, 2012) emphasize the need for nurses with master's degrees to be competent in acquiring, appraising, implementing, and evaluating best evidence for nursing practice.

Between 2010 and 2012, our large university school of nursing undertook a major curriculum revision to align graduate curricula for advanced practice nursing, education, and administration tracks with newly revised curricular standards published by the AACN and NONPF. In this chapter, we identify essential evidence-based practice (EBP) concepts, share the development of an EBP core course for MSN students, describe course delivery for online and face-to-face educational environments, and summarize selected module assignments. We identify useful web-based strategies for the implementation of student learning and engagement with EBP.

## BACKGROUND

EBP has been defined as "the conscientious, explicit, and judicious use of current best evidence in making decisions about the care of individual patients" (Sackett, Rosenberg, Gray, Haynes, & Richardson, 1996, p. 71). Previous MSN core courses did not prepare students with the skill sets necessary to assess, evaluate, and apply EBP. In the newly designed curriculum, students take a research course that incorporates statistics the first semester and Evidence for Advanced Nursing Practice the second semester.

The EBP course was designed to promote student review, critique, and application of EBP in practice. It focuses on developing an understanding of evidence-based conceptual models and approaches to nursing practice, employing relevant strategies and tools in an effort to link research, evidence, and practice. Four multipart learning modules were designed to achieve the expected learning outcomes for each course objective. Module titles, objectives, and assignments for the course are listed in Table 9.1.

## THE LEARNING MODULES

Module 1 introduces students to EBP history, core principles (research application, clinical expertise, and patient preference), and use in healthcare environments. Students construct a correctly formatted PICOT question (Melnyk & Fineout-Overholt, 2011), where *P* represents the patient population, *I* represents either the intervention or an issue to be addressed, *C* represents the comparison intervention or group, *O* represents the outcome, and *T* represents the time frame. Writing a correctly worded, searchable, and answerable question is essential for guiding students through the EBP process and locating the EBP guideline most suited to the client's problem. To find an EBP intervention/practice guideline as a potential answer for the PICOT question, students search one or more of the university's online databases.

In Module 2, the focus shifts from using and identifying evidence to ensuring that evidence is functional and valuable for application in the practice arena. Students use the AGREE II Assessment tool to critically appraise a selected guideline across seven domains for determining its fit with the client's problem for a selected practice setting (Brouwers et al., 2010). With this tool, the student can assess the rigor of the method used in developing the practice guideline and document its internal and external validity as a basis for recommending its use (National Collaborating Centre for Methods and Tools, 2011).

As students critically appraise the guideline, they develop a beginning understanding of the measurement of risk concepts, odds ratios, and confidence intervals. To demonstrate understanding of risk concepts, students select the correct responses to quiz items. In preparation for taking the quiz, students read and interpret key measurements of risk concepts contained in an assigned EBP article.

In Module 3, students are introduced to several commonly used EBP implementation models and determine their appropriateness for application in a selected practice setting for their original PICOT question. Some models fit best for inpatient or outpatient practice settings, whereas others are robust enough for use in educational and administrative domains. Students also explore ethical principles inherent in applying evidence by using classical ethics theory, including beneficence, nonmaleficence, justice, and autonomy, as well as 15 subcategories outlined by Melnyk and Fineout-Overholt (2011). Discussions take place online in discussion board postings or face-to-face courses. Each student serves as a moderator for the discussion of one complex ethical dilemma and the integration of core ethical principles.

## TABLE 9.1

## Evidence for Advanced Nursing Practice Objectives and Assignments by Module

| Module | Objectives | Assignments |
|---|---|---|
| *Module 1* <br> Exploring EBP | The student will: <br> 1. Analyze the historical development of EBP. <br> 2. Critically appraise elements of EBP. <br> 3. Examine steps in the process to use evidence as the basis for nursing practice. <br> 4. Implement strategies to optimize the search for evidence to support nursing practice. | • Literature and website reading <br> • Identification of burning clinical questions <br> • Written PICOT question |
| *Module 2* <br> Appraising the Evidence | 1. Analyze the strength of the evidence as an intervention. <br> 2. Evaluate types of bias affecting the validity of a study. <br> 3. Determine magnitude of effect. <br> 4. Determine the strength of association (i.e., ARR, RRR, NNT, OR, and CI). <br> 5. Analyze EBP guidelines for utility, validity, and reliability using the AGREE II tool. | • Literature/website reading <br> • EBP statistics quiz <br> • Selection of EBP guideline for best fit with PICOT <br> • AGREE II tool assessment of selected EBP guideline <br> • Three-page summary of assessment results and application recommendation(s) |
| *Module 3* <br> Models/Ethics of EBP | 1. Evaluate different EBP models to determine suitability for use in different practice settings. <br> 2. Integrate ethical principles into EBP applications. | • Literature/website reading <br> • Response to ethical-based question (500 words) <br> • Compare/contrast 2 EBP models |

*(continued)*

| TABLE 9.1 |
|---|

## Evidence for Advanced Nursing Practice Objectives and Assignments by Module (*Continued*)

| Module | Objectives | Assignments |
|---|---|---|
| *Module 4*<br>Implementing EBP | 1. Appraise current knowledge and practice related to a defined PICOT question.<br><br>2. Use established criteria to critically appraise evidence.<br><br>3. Recommend change/improvement of current practice, policy, or procedure based on evidence.<br><br>4. Propose plan for changing or reinforcing recommended practice.<br><br>5. Work effectively as a contributing team member to the group project. | • Critical appraisal of evidence process for 5 EBP studies<br><br>• Five-page paper addressing PICOT, critical appraisal of the evidence, and recommendations for change in clinical practice (group project) |

EBP, evidence-based practice; ARR, absolute risk reduction; RRR, relative risk reduction; NNT, number needed to treat; OR, odds ratio; CI, confidence interval.

The purpose of Module 4 is to incorporate learning from previous modules into a small (two-person) group project. Students use the principles and context of EBP to develop a beginning practice model based on a PICOT question developed in Module 1. A healthcare practice intervention, policy, or procedure is evaluated, and a recommendation for change or improvement is proposed. If a change or improvement is not needed, a thorough explanation must be provided for why the existing intervention, policy, or procedure represents best evidence.

Narrative components of the assignment include the PICOT question, critical appraisal of the evidence, and the proposed change in clinical practice. The strength of the evidence (research, patient/family preferences and values, and clinical expertise) is evaluated and serves as the basis for recommendations for a current healthcare practice, policy, or procedure revision.

## CHALLENGES

The new core course has been offered every semester since spring 2012. Although no major problems were encountered, several challenges implementing the course online have been identified, including the following:

- The daunting volume of information about available EBP, along with an overwhelming number of textbooks and an excessive number of external resources
- Links to online resources in modules not active for the entire semester that often require the purchase of a subscription
- The need to assist students in understanding the use of statistics to report health associations and outcomes, including measures of risk, odds ratios, and confidence intervals
- The limited translation of newly learned EBP assessment and evaluation skill sets to successive courses

Strategies developed by faculty and students to successfully address the challenges include the following:

- Selecting the most current edition of the Melynk and Fineout-Overholt (2011) text has helped to address the challenge of the daunting volume of EBP information, as faculty have found it to be focused on EBP that is appropriate for each MSN track (APRN, educator, and administrator), as well as useful for MSN student learning and the implementation of MSN graduate roles (APRN, educator, administrator).
- Reducing the number of external links and providing faculty guidance in accessing resources through the university library has addressed the challenge of online link malfunctions.
- The use of statistics to report health associations has been addressed by student "word of mouth" (current students have been forewarned to study risk concepts because all are used in successive courses) and the development of a one-page resource guide for use in the EBP course and successive courses.
- Limited translation and applicability of the newly acquired EBP assessment and evaluation skill sets has been addressed by faculty via the development of EBP assignments in successive courses.

## OUTCOMES AND CONCLUSION

Several valuable outcomes have been achieved. A brief listing follows:

- Increased application of the EBP concepts in successive courses
- Use of the AGREE II tool by one or more students asked to revise policies and procedures at work (self-report to faculty)
- Building on a Module 4 project in successive course(s) and applying it to a population focus in a community
- Acceptance of two student projects for presentation at the 42nd Sigma Theta Tau International Research Congress

Faculty worked diligently in reviewing and revising the course to improve learning experiences and increase the achievement level of learning outcomes. A brief list of improvement strategies designed to date includes the following:

- Use of a short statistics quiz to motivate "serious" focus on learning measurement statistics (the quiz contributes 5 percent of the course grade; insufficient points can cause course failure; the quiz can precipitate "math fear" anxieties)
- Reduction of course content from "nice to know" or "everything you ever wanted to know" about EBP ("content creep") to essentials of EBP concepts and principles
- Increasing all MSN faculty comfort with incorporating EBP concepts in assignments for other applicable courses (faculty development sessions about what EBP is and is not, how to add measurement statistics and the use of the critique and evaluation skill set to applicable course assignments)
- Decreasing the student tendency to isolate course content/skills to one course (inclusion of EBP application in assignments for successive courses; integrating EBP concepts and principles into successive course class discussion boards)
- Faculty discussion of how EBP principles and concepts can be integrated into assignments in other courses during the curriculum review process

Increasing emphasis on EBP concepts and principles across the MSN curriculum is essential for preparing graduates as critical appraisers of evidence and not merely EBP guideline followers. The new core course demonstrates effective teaching of EBP in a distance or classroom setting while producing evidence translation from the early stages of PICOT question development to evidence selection and appraisal, including consideration of practice-based and ethical issues prior to the dissemination and implementation phase of evidence integration.

## *References*

American Association of Colleges of Nursing (AACN). (2011). *The essentials of master's education in nursing.* Washington, DC: Author.

Brouwers, M. C., Kho, M. E., Browman, G. P., Burgers, J. S., Cluzeau, F., Feder, G., et al., for the AGREE Next Steps Consortium. (2010). AGREE II: Advancing guideline development, reporting and evaluation in health care. *Canadian Medical Association Journal, 182*(18), E839–E842.

Melnyk, B., & Fineout-Overholt, E. (2011). *Evidence-based practice in nursing and healthcare: A guide to best practice.* Philadelphia, PA: Lippincott Williams & Wilkins.

National Collaborating Centre for Methods and Tools. (2011, updated November 1, 2013). *Critically appraising practice guidelines: The AGREE II instrument.* Hamilton, ON, Canada: McMaster University. Available from www.nccmt.ca/registry/view/eng/100.html

National Organization of Nurse Practitioner Faculties (NONPF). (2012). *Nurse practitioner core competencies.* Washington, DC: Author.

Sackett, D. L., Rosenberg, W. M., Gray, J. A., Haynes, R. B., & Richardson, W. S. (1996). Evidence based medicine: What it is and what it isn't. *British Medical Journal, 312*(7023), 71–72.

# 10

# Facilitating Undergraduate Nursing Students' Appraisal of Evidence

**Margaret J. Bull,** PhD, RN

Evidence-based practice (EBP) has been defined as a framework for clinical practice that integrates best available scientific evidence with clinical expertise, and patient preferences and values to make decisions about health care (Melnyk, Fineout-Overholt, Stillwell, & Williamson, 2009). Although there are various definitions of EBP, the common elements include integrating the best available evidence, clinician expertise, and patient preferences and values in making decisions about health care with the goal of achieving high-quality, cost-effective care (Institute of Medicine [IOM], 2012; Schmidt & Brown, 2012).

## EVIDENCE-BASED PRACTICE IN UNDERGRADUATE NURSING CURRICULA

Forces within and outside the discipline of nursing provide an impetus for teaching EBP in undergraduate nursing curricula. The *Essentials for Baccalaureate Education* (American Association of Colleges of Nursing, 2008) states that graduates of baccalaureate programs are expected to be able to appraise and integrate evidence in practice. The IOM recommended evidence-based decision-making as one of the five core competencies for healthcare professionals (IOM, 2001) and later recommended that education programs teach healthcare professionals ways of accessing, managing, and applying evidence in providing patient care (IOM, 2012). Consequently, nurse educators are faced with the challenge of teaching undergraduate students to appraise evidence and consider how the evidence might be applied in clinical practice.

## The Challenge of Identifying Article Type

Typically, the undergraduate research course in a curriculum is charged with teaching students to appraise evidence. Although undergraduate research courses place emphasis on appraisal of research studies, the evidence pyramid includes other types of articles, such as expert opinion, practice guidelines, and editorials. Thus, students need to be able to recognize the type of article being appraised. Undergraduate students often find identifying the type of article a difficult task even after receiving an orientation to database searching by a librarian and participating in class discussion about the types of articles (Meeker, Jones, & Flanagan, 2008). Furthermore, faculty teaching clinical courses comment that students who have completed an undergraduate research course have difficulty identifying the type of article selected for clinical conference discussion.

## The "What Type of Article Is It?" Grid

This chapter describes the use of a grid titled "What Type of Article Is It?" to help junior-level nursing students recognize the type of article being appraised. The grid (Table 10.1) was provided to 59 students enrolled in an undergraduate research course during the first class session. Students were told that the grid would be used in class for journal club discussions, and they were encouraged to use the grid in appraising articles for their evidence-based project. The common cues for each type of article were listed in the columns below the article type. For instance, the cues in Table 10.1 for a qualitative study include the use of research headings (aims, methods, sample, findings), the collection of words/narrative data, a sample from one study, the use of observation or semistructured interviews to collect data, and direct quotes from study participants. A copy of the grid was available to students throughout the course on the online course management system.

As the course progressed, the types of articles discussed in the journal clubs during class moved up the evidence pyramid from expert opinion and single qualitative studies to correlational studies, experimental, and randomized controlled trials. The question ("What type of article is it?") was posed for each journal club discussion, and cues to article type were identified. For the final class project, groups of five to seven students worked together to appraise evidence about strategies to reduce medication errors in patients who were hospitalized. Each group completed a table that included the citation for each student's article, purpose of the study, type of article, level of evidence, method, results, and recommendations. In addition, each group gave an oral presentation summarizing the article types, levels of evidence, similarities and differences in findings, and their evaluation of the relevance of the findings for clinical practice. The majority of students (95 percent) in the research course accurately identified the type of article for their projects. In contrast, only 70 percent of students in the previous semester accurately identified the type of article without using the "What Type of Article Is It?" grid. Moreover, 52 of the 59 students enrolled in the research course were simultaneously enrolled in a course on the essentials of gerontological nursing, which required students to select and appraise a research report on delirium, dementia, or depression. This was an end-of-course assignment with an expectation that students would apply what they had learned in the research course about appraising studies in completing this assignment. The majority of students (97 percent) accurately identified the type of article. Two students, who were not successful in accurately identifying the article type, did not use the grid in appraising their article because they thought that the grid should only apply to the research course.

# TABLE 10.1

## What Type of Article Is It?

| | Literature Reviews | | | Quantitative Studies | | | |
| Expert Opinion | Integrative | Meta-synthesis | Meta-analysis | Descriptive | Correlational or Comparative | Experiment | Qualitative Studies |
|---|---|---|---|---|---|---|---|
| Absence of research headings | Absence of research headings | Research headings (i.e., aim, methods, sample, findings, discussion) | Research headings (i.e., aim, methods, sample, findings, discussion) | Research headings (i.e., aim, methods, sample, findings, discussion) | Research headings (i.e., aim, methods, sample, findings, discussion) | Research headings (i.e., aim, methods, sample, findings, discussion) | Research headings (i.e., aim, methods, sample, findings, discussion) |
| Often written in first person (e.g., "I" or "we") | Often written in third person | Word data | Numeric data | Numeric data | Numeric data | Numeric data Describes intervention or manipulation of IV | Words or narrative data |
| Absence of sample | Focused topic Reviews theories and/or research papers | Sample consists of number of qualitative studies with similar focus | Sample consists of number of quantitative studies with similar variables | Sample for one study | Sample for one study | Sample for one study | Sample for one study |

(continued)

# TABLE 10.1

## What Type of Article Is It? (*Continued*)

| Expert Opinion | Literature Reviews | | | Quantitative Studies | | | Qualitative Studies |
|---|---|---|---|---|---|---|---|
| | Integrative | Meta-synthesis | Meta-analysis | Descriptive | Correlational or Comparative | Experiment | |
| Absence of data collection | Published works | Number of articles retrieved Published and unpublished | Number of articles retrieved Published and unpublished | Data collection instruments (e.g., scales, numbers) | Data collection instruments (e.g., scales, numbers) | Data collection instruments (e.g., scales, numbers) | Description of semistructured interview or observation (e.g., "Tell me what it is like…") |
| Summary of ideas or topic | Summary of knowledge on topic | Synthesize findings in words | Statistics Estimate effect | Descriptive statistics such as frequencies | Inferential statistics such as correlations, regression | Inferential statistics comparing groups (e.g., t-test) | Verbatim exemplars |
| Absence of tables with data | Absence of table listing articles | Tables list articles | Tables list articles | Tables of numeric findings | Tables of numeric findings | Tables of numeric findings | Tables with exemplars |

# CONCLUSION

In summary, undergraduate students need guidance in learning to identify the type of article they are appraising and in applying knowledge acquired in a research course to clinically focused courses. The use of the "What Type of Article Is It?" grid contributed to students' ability to accurately identify the types of articles used in the final class project for the research course and for an assignment in a gerontological nursing course.

## References

American Association of Colleges of Nursing. (2008). *The essentials of baccalaureate education for professional nursing*. Washington, DC: Author.

Institute of Medicine. (2001). *Crossing the quality chasm: A new health system for the 21st century*. Washington, DC: National Academies Press.

Institute of Medicine. (2012). *Best care at lower cost*. Washington, DC: National Academies Press.

Meeker, M., Jones, J. M., & Flanagan, N. A. (2008). Teaching undergraduate nursing research from an evidence-based practice perspective. *Journal of Nursing Education, 47*(8), 376–379.

Melnyk, B., Fineout-Overholt, E., Stillwell, S., & Williamson, K. M. (2009). Igniting a spirit of inquiry: An essential foundation to evidence-based practice. *American Journal of Nursing, 109*(11), 49–52.

Schmidt, N. A., & Brown, J. M. (2012). *Evidence-based practice for nurses: Appraisal and application of research*. Sudbury, MA: Jones & Bartlett Learning.

# 11

# Implementing a Pediatric Camp Clinical for Pre-Licensure Education

**Desiree Hensel,** PhD, RN, PNCS-BC, CNE
**Claire Malinowski,** BSN, RN
**Patricia A. Watts,** DNP, RN, CNS, PNP-BC

Pediatrics has been reported to be the most stressful rotation for many students (Lassche, Al-Qaaydeh, Macintosh, & Black, 2013; Oermann & Lukomski, 2001). With a lack of adequate clinical sites threatening the quality of pediatric education (Bultas, 2011), and the pediatric unit of our rural hospital frequently subject to low patient census, our traditional nursing students had limited exposure to children with medical needs.

Leaders in nursing education have called for a greater emphasis on the use of community-based clinical sites (Benner, Sutphen, Leonard, & Day, 2010). Although camp settings have been proposed as such an alternative for pediatric education, allowing students to care for children with a wide variety of needs in a relaxed environment (Broussard & Meaux, 2007; Schmidt, 2007), summer is the prime time for such camps to operate. Our challenge was to create a camp clinical during the fall to spring academic year that met our pediatric course's minimum requirement of 56 hours of clinical education.

## CREATING THE CAMP CLINICAL

In fall 2010, we piloted a pediatric clinical rotation in a wilderness setting at our university-affiliated camp. The regular course instructor for the junior-level BSN course was a pediatric nurse practitioner who worked summers at that camp. After meeting with the camp administrators, we were invited to bring students to two weekend fall retreats offered for children, ages 8 to 18 years, with disabilities and chronic conditions, such as being wheelchair bound or having a cognitive impairment. In the camp application material, parents were advised that nursing students may be caring for their children while at camp.

We decided to offer this clinical opportunity to one cohort of 10 students, with 5 students at each retreat. However, one retreat was canceled, and the decision was made to send all 10 students to the remaining camp with 21 campers. (One student became ill and could not attend.)

Students were recruited through an email sent prior to the start of the semester. The response was highly favorable, with 16 out of 20 eligible students expressing interest in the alternative practicum.

To prepare for the experience, the students spent 4 hours with the instructor in the nursing learning resource center (NLRC) becoming educated in pediatric nursing skills; an additional 4 hours were dedicated to high-fidelity simulation. On the Friday of the retreat, students attended a camp orientation.

Students were divided among cabin groups where they lived, working beside experienced counselors and providing needed medical care for the campers. During waking hours, the students attended planned camp activities, administered medications and treatments, and assisted with activities of daily living. At night, the students rotated the duty of hourly rounds and provided needed care, such as turning campers and changing incontinence undergarments. The instructor also stayed on-site around the clock to provide supervision.

All skills performed were documented on a course inventory, and an instructor-led postconference was held at the end of camp. Students were then asked to submit a reflective entry of their thoughts and feelings to an online forum, including what they did or did not learn about pediatric nursing and how they met course objectives. Students were also asked to provide examples, in a subsequent forum entry, of how camp had helped them attain knowledge, skills, and attitudes consistent with Quality and Safety for Nursing (QSEN) competencies (Cronenwett et al., 2007).

## FOCUS GROUP EVALUATION

Institutional review board approval was obtained to conduct an audio-taped focus group session. All students gave informed consent to analyze their work and volunteered to participate in the focus group, which was led by a senior nursing honors student. Here are the main lessons we learned.

## Lesson 1: The Camp Environment Supported Patient-Centered Care

All students were able to give examples of how they met both course and QSEN competencies in the online forums and on the course self-evaluation. The strongest theme from the forums and focus groups was that students were able to gain a greater appreciation of the multiple dimensions of patient-centered care. Specific QSEN attitudes identified by Cronenwett et al. (2007) that students expressed included:

- Value seeing through patients' eyes.
- Respect and encourage the expression of patient preferences and needs.
- Value patients' expertise with their own health.
- Seek learning opportunities with patients.
- Respect patient preference for engagement in care.
- Recognize personally held attitudes about working with patients from different backgrounds.
- Appreciate the role of the nurse in the relief of suffering.

As an example, one student spoke of putting the campers' usual routines and needs before her own. Another stated that she wanted to help the campers, to the extent possible, maintain their daily routine to make the camp experience comfortable. Some students discussed how they promoted independence by only assisting if a camper requested help. Others reported benefiting from the opportunity to develop their communication skills.

Several students related that by experiencing the daily lives and challenges of individuals with chronic health concerns, they were able to gain a sense of empathy. One student shared that the campers' positive attitudes made all students value their own lives more and not take as much for granted.

## Lesson 2: Students Felt Supported and Relaxed But Could Have Had More Preparation

Students performed a variety of nursing skills, many of which were not typically performed at our rural hospital, including gastrostomy tube feedings, Mace stoma care, nebulizer treatments, and catheterizations. The campers' relaxed attitudes about the procedures lessened the nursing students' tension and made them more confident about performing new skills. One student commented, "They were not nervous about it, so I thought, why should I be?"

The students spoke of the abundance of support they received from the counselors, the staff, and their instructor, noting that they did not always receive such support in the hospital setting. They felt comfortable asking questions and did not feel as pressed for time as they typically felt in the hospital. Teamwork was a major component of the weekend. Adhering to the camp policy that no one should ever be alone, students worked collaboratively to organize and prioritize care for their campers. All participants agreed that the camp reinforced their decision to choose nursing as a career.

Students did, however, state that they would have liked more preparation. Many campers had unusual conditions, and the students suggested that having a list of potential diagnoses to research before attending the camp could be helpful. In addition, the time in the NLRC could have been more focused on the procedures and skills specific to camp versus general pediatrics. For instance, camp procedures for verifying patient identity included reading an armband and comparing it to medication cards. This differed greatly from hospital bar code scanning and could have been practiced in a simulation. Finally, exposing students to the care of Monti and Mace stomas and practice with administering enteral feedings would better prepare them for this experience.

## Lesson 3: Scheduling Was a Barrier

The cancellation of one of the two scheduled retreats due to lack of interest by campers happened at a time when it was impossible to reschedule the students to the hospital setting. In addition, we were unable to allow the student who missed the retreat because of illness to make up her clinical hours during the semester. The student was given an incomplete and had to return during the summer to complete the make-up experience at camp with the instructor.

## CONCLUSION

Students will never have identical clinical experiences, and our institution maintains that as long as students meet course competencies, different sites and approaches can be used. The course self-evaluation showed that students from the camp group were able to articulate the ways they met each competency. Feedback was positive from the campers, staff, and students. We found the camp experience to be superior to the hospital environment in many ways, but especially for teaching the QSEN competency of patient-centered care.

Because the students slept with the campers in the cabins and attended to their needs at night, we counted all hours at camp as clinical time. Still, we were concerned that working only with special needs school-aged children and adolescents limited the students' exposure to the greater pediatric population, including younger children. To gain a broader pediatric experience, the decision was made that future camp cohorts would include some clinical hours at a pediatric primary provider's office. We also decided that future cohorts would receive a more targeted orientation with a list of potential camper diagnoses.

With 60 students a year enrolled in our pediatric course and the limited camp dates during the school year, our institution will only have the opportunity to offer this option to a small portion of students. We have added a summer camp pediatric elective to our curriculum but have had limited interest because our students typically seek paid internships in the summer. However, there is a growing imperative to offer more summer classes and to graduate students in an accelerated time frame. As we plan for a year-round cohort, we hope to move our pediatric course to the summer to take full advantage of the numerous pediatric specialty camps.

### References

Benner, P., Sutphen, M., Leonard, V., & Day, L. (2010). *Educating nurses: A call for radical transformation.* San Francisco, CA: Jossey-Bass.

Broussard, L., & Meaux, J. (2007). Camp nursing: Rewards and challenges. *Pediatric Nursing, 33*(3), 238–242.

Bultas, M. W. (2011). Enhancing the pediatric undergraduate nursing curriculum through simulation. *Journal of Pediatric Nursing, 26*(3), 224–229.

Cronenwett, L., Sherwood, G., Barnsteiner, J., Disch, J., Johnson, J., Mitchell, P., et al. (2007). Quality and safety education for nurses. *Nursing Outlook, 55*(3), 122–131.

Lassche, M., Al-Qaaydeh, S., Macintosh, C. I., & Black, M. (2013). Identifying changes in comfort and worry among pediatric nursing students following clinical rotations. *Journal of Pediatric Nursing, 28*(1), 48–54.

Oermann, M. H., & Lukomski, A. P. (2001). Experiences of students in pediatric nursing clinical courses. *Journal for Specialists in Pediatric Nursing, 6*(2), 65–72.

Schmidt, L. (2007). Camp nursing: Innovative opportunities for nursing students to work with children. *Nurse Educator, 32*(6), 246–250.

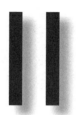

# The NLN Center for Assessment and Evaluation

# 12

# Improving Nursing Students' Academic Performance Through The Exam Analysis

**Vaneta M. Condon,** PhD, MSN, RN
**Earline M. W. Miller,** PhD, MPH, RN
**Iris Mamier,** PhD, MSN, RN
**Grenith J. Zimmerman,** PhD
**Barbara L. Ninan,** MN, RN

Nursing faculty often struggle to find strategies to help frustrated and over-whelmed at-risk nursing students pass nursing courses and succeed academically (Poorman, Mastorovitch, & Webb, 2011). Higher than average attrition rates have been reported for minority students (Davidhizar & Shearer, 2005), who often face serious barriers to their academic success (Igbo et al., 2011). Other at-risk groups include nontraditional nursing students who may juggle family responsibilities while going to nursing school, commuters, and students who work more than 16 hours per week (Jeffreys, 2012).

When compared to students who maintain strong passing grades, at-risk students may have inadequate test-taking skills (English & Gordon, 2004) and greater anxiety (McGann & Thompson, 2008). At-risk students who underperform are more likely to have inadequate learning strategies, are less likely to seek help (Rheinheimer, Grace-Odeleye, Francois, & Kusorgbor, 2010), have lower levels of motivation (Balduf, 2009), and may have less cognitive behavioral engagement (Rachal, Daigle, & Rachal, 2007).

The early work on student attrition focused on the belief that the student, not the institution, was the problem (Tinto, 2006, 2012). Academic failure was blamed on the student's lack of ability and motivation. Tinto (2012) countered this blame the victim mentality by arguing that the institution is partially responsible for the continued inequity of graduation rates among minority students. However, although it is the responsibility of the institution to create an academic and social environment that leads to success, faculty are often at a loss in knowing how to specifically support students academically. The Exam Analysis© (TEA) is an intervention strategy that can encourage student academic success.

The purpose of this chapter is to describe TEA, which is a diagnostic and prescriptive program designed to help students learn from incorrect answers and restrategize after a nursing exam, and to evaluate the effect of participating in TEA by comparing exam scores before TEA with final exam scores after TEA. TEA is used to improve exam performance for nursing students who are at risk for failure and those who are underperforming. However, the focus of this study is on at-risk students who scored below 85 percent in Fundamentals of Professional Nursing (Fundamentals) and/or Medical-Surgical Nursing I (Med-Surg I).

# BACKGROUND

TEA is a diagnostic and prescriptive educational strategy developed to assist nursing students in achieving academic success. A student who desires to improve nursing exam scores meets with an RN Learning Assistance Program (LAP) facilitator to review and identify reasons for incorrect answers selected by the student on a nursing exam. Incorrect answers are then categorized into five problem areas (Lack of Knowledge, English Language Skills, Exam Panic, Exam Skills, and Other) that are then further divided into subcategories. Following TEA, diagnoses are made by totaling the scores and providing a percentage from each of the categories that accounted for the missed questions. The prescriptive portion of TEA is achieved by providing specific intervention strategies that focus on each of the five categories. An essential ingredient of TEA results from the one-on-one support that the student receives from the LAP facilitator.

TEA process was developed in the mid-1980s in response to nursing faculty's concerns that some students who did well in clinical nursing still failed their nursing exams. In an effort to assist at-risk students in improving their grades on exams and regaining their self-confidence after experiencing failure, two faculty members reviewed incorrect exam answers with these students and identified possible reasons why individual questions were answered incorrectly. These reasons fell into the five categories that became the basis for the development of TEA worksheet. As faculty used this worksheet with nursing students, they further divided the five categories into 16 subcategories (Figure 12.1).

The diagnostic procedure of TEA is outlined in Box 12.1. There are 10 steps that make up TEA procedure. The prescriptive procedure (Intervention Strategies to Improve Exam Performance) was developed after reviewing nursing research literature that focused on intervention strategies for each of the five categories (Box 12.2). TEA encompasses student and facilitator researched and agreed upon specific interventions to help students improve in the areas identified.

TEA interventions are supplemented with required workshops and seminars to increase study skill knowledge. Topics include reading textbooks, time management, note taking, and exam-taking skills. In addition, TEA facilitators model the desired behavior, apply critical thinking, encourage problem solving, recommend specific study skills, promote weekly study groups, and refer the student to the LAP for additional help. Properly utilized, TEA is a strong example of an effective intervention that represents faculty support.

Sometimes English language problems do not become apparent until diagnosed during TEA. At this time, the facilitator seeks to determine the extent of the language barrier. If language is the major cause of failure on an exam, it will be recommended that the student take remedial English language classes. In addition, students with extremely limited English language proficiency are referred to a university-based English as a second

**OBJECTIVE EXAM ANALYSIS WORKSHEET**

Student _____    Course _____    Exam _____

   Grade _____    Date _____

| Test missed item | Lack of Knowledge | | | | | English Skills | | | | Exam Panic | | | | Exam Skills | | | | | | Other | | ANALYSIS RESULTS |
|---|---|---|---|---|---|---|---|---|---|---|---|---|---|---|---|---|---|---|---|---|---|---|
| | Reading/textbook | Inadequate notes | Application of knowledge | Poor retention | Other | Reading comprehension | Reading speed | Vocabulary | Other | Decreased concentration | Mental block | Forgot to use exam techniques | Other | Did not focus on what question asked | Failed to consider options carefully (True, False, ?, etc.) | Poor use of time | Changed answer | Carelessness/clerical error | Other | Math | Other | |
| | | | | | | | | | | | | | | | | | | | | | | |
| | | | | | | | | | | | | | | | | | | | | | | |
| | | | | | | | | | | | | | | | | | | | | | | |
| | | | | | | | | | | | | | | | | | | | | | | |
| | | | | | | | | | | | | | | | | | | | | | | |
| | | | | | | | | | | | | | | | | | | | | | | |
| | | | | | | | | | | | | | | | | | | | | | | |
| | | | | | | | | | | | | | | | | | | | | | | |
| # | | | | | | | | | | | | | | | | | | | | | | |
| % | | | | | | | | | | | | | | | | | | | | | | |
| % Total | | | | | | | | | | | | | | | | | | | | | | |

**FIGURE 12.1** The Exam Analysis Worksheet. From Loma Linda University School of Nursing, Learning Assistance Program. Copyright 1986, 2006, Loma Linda University.

language (ESL) language immersion program. These programs often include speaking, reading, writing, vocabulary, use of vocabulary idioms, pronunciation, grammar, and study skills.

Once implemented, the faculty soon noted an increase in the exam passing rate when students used TEA interventions. In fact, students from other surrounding schools of nursing (SONs) came to the Loma Linda University SON for TEA interventions. TEA has been used extensively at other SONs in the United States, Canada, and other countries. TEA has also been shared with nursing educators at conferences and reported in the nursing literature (Caputi & Engelman, 2008; Condon & Drew, 1995). In 1995, one study reported that 97 percent of the 105 nursing students surveyed indicated improved grades and increased feelings of self-worth following participation in TEA (Condon & Drew).

---

## BOX 12.1

## The Exam Analysis Procedure

The following steps make up the exam analysis procedure:

1. The student and instructor/learning facilitator become aware that the student has a problem with taking exams.
2. The student requests an exam analysis.
3. The student and instructor/learning facilitator who is doing the analysis discuss the LAP Summary of Exam Techniques for Multiple Choice Questions (see Box 12.3).
4. The student and instructor/learning facilitator go over each question which the student missed on the exam. The student uses the exam techniques to answer these questions. (The student does not look at his former answer or at the correct answer on the answer key.)
5. The student and instructor/learning facilitator identify the main category and specific problem or contributing factor for why the student missed each question.
6. The instructor/learning facilitator records why each item was missed on the exam analysis worksheet.
7. The instructor/learning facilitator totals the number of items missed and the percentages for each specific problem and each main category.
8. Suggested interventions are developed with input from the student and recorded on the Suggestions to Improve Exam Performance checklist (see Box 12.2).
9. A copy of the exam analysis is given to the student, and another is retained in the student's record.
10. Follow-up appointments (or referrals) for help with exam skills, tutoring, counseling and evaluation of progress are made.

From Loma Linda University School of Nursing, Learning Assistance Program. Copyright 1986, 2006, Loma Linda University.

An unpublished anonymous 2008 survey of 76 nursing students who participated in TEA ranked the following three outcomes as most important. In order of importance, they were (1) improved knowledge of subject matter through use of better study habits/skills (45.9 percent), (2) improved exam-taking strategies (27.0 percent), and (3) decreased anxiety (18.9 percent). Participants also ranked the three most important exam-taking strategies as follows: (1) identifying key words while reading the question (64.9 percent), (2) thinking through and writing down their own answer before reading the answer options on the exam (21.6 percent), and (3) eliminating wrong answers and then choosing the best answer (21.6 percent). Student comments regarding what encouraged them the most included:

- "Going over the test and analyzing what I did wrong."
- "The idea that I could come up with the answer before looking at the options, and if I wasn't sure, I could use my strategies to help me find the answer."
- "[TEA] lowers the level of anxiety during the exam & improves self-confidence."

## BOX 12.2

## Checklist: Suggestions to Improve Exam Performance

**Priority #_____ Lack of Knowledge of Subject Matter**

____ 1. Use study guide/objective/specific class guidelines to identify important content while reading textbook.

____ 2. Write out key points from #1 and use for later review.

____ 3. Take careful notes during class.

____ 4. As soon as possible <u>after class</u> and at <u>the end of each week</u> review, #2 & #3 from above.

____ 5. Participate in study group each week.

____ 6. Use NCLEX-RN review books to review important content and to practice application on review questions.

____ 7. Predict exam questions — use these for group review.

____ 8. Schedule time to review each lecture carefully before exam.

____ 9. Note weak areas such as Pathophysiology, Medication, side effects, lab values, etc.

**Priority # _____ Exam-Taking Skills**

____ 1. Read each question carefully and <u>underline or circle key words</u>.

____ 2. Give your <u>own answer</u> (write down a few words <u>BEFORE</u> looking at choices given on exam).

____ 3. Mark each answer choices as T, F, ?, ?T, ?F.

____ 4. Choose the best answer based on what you learned in this class.

____ 5. <u>Don't</u> change your answer unless you <u>know why</u> the first answer is wrong. (Never change an answer just because you <u>feel uncertain</u>.

____ 6. <u>Practice application</u> of knowledge to <u>case studies/NCLEX-RN review questions</u>.

**Priority # _____ English Language/Vocabulary**

____ 1. Look up vocabulary terms/new words identified in reading assignment, lecture, study group, etc.

____ 2. Write out the meanings of these words/pronunciations and use them in a sentence on flash cards, or in a notebook (using 2-column format).

____ 3. Drill on these words several times each week.

____ 4. If you don't understand an exam question or answer choice, ask the instructor for clarification.

**Priority # _____ Exam Anxiety**

____ 1. <u>Overprepare for exam</u> so that you feel <u>confident</u> about your knowledge.

____ 2. Use <u>exam-taking skills</u> discussed in LAP—this helps you think logically one step at a time.

____ 3. Use positive self-talk (i.e., "I know these concepts, I am going to do well on this exam.")

____ 4. Don't spend too long on a difficult question. This lowers your confidence and ↑ anxiety. Read it carefully 2×, guess, and move on to easier questions. Come back later if you have time.

____ 5. Pray that God will help you feel calm and help you remember what you have learned and help you apply knowledge and exam skills.

____ 6. Practice relaxation techniques (deep breathing, etc.) so you can use them p.r.n.

- "Knowing that someone was there to help me understand what went wrong on my test."
- "[TEA] gave me the strength and encouragement to continue my nursing career."

Each of the five categories on TEA worksheet (Lack of Knowledge, English Language Skills, Exam Panic, Exam Skills, and Other) is documented in the nursing literature as a possible problem area for nursing students. The literature review that follows focuses on these five categories and provides selected interventions for each. This evidence established from the literature then forms the basis for the prescriptive part of TEA as an educational tool.

## REVIEW OF THE LITERATURE
## Lack of Knowledge

One of the major problems related to poor academic success in nursing is a lack of knowledge of the subject matter. This has been found to be related to several factors. Low pre-admission test scores in science, reading, and total Test of Essential Academic Skills were found by Wolkowitz and Kelly (2010) to predict poor academic performance. In addition, low scores in critical thinking (Ellis, 2006; McGann & Thompson, 2008; Rachal et al., 2007; Thomas & Baker, 2011) and low grades in nursing courses (Fike, McCall, Rachal, Smith, & Lockman, 2010; Pitt, Powis, Levett-Jones, & Hunter, 2012; Pryjmachuk, Easton, & Lockwood, 2009) predict low achievement in nursing school.

Other factors that contribute to a lack of knowledge include inadequate preparatory education and poor study skills (Hendry & Farley, 2006; Igbo et al., 2011; Pauk & Owens, 2011). Learning process research reviewed by August-Brady (2005) found that students who use deep learning approaches and utilize metacognitive strategies enjoy greater academic success. Raising the admission requirements for Texas Women's University by requiring higher scores on the critical thinking analysis portion of the nursing entrance exam increased the number of students who successfully graduated from first-level nursing courses (Ellis, 2006).

Poor learning strategies and deficits in critical thinking continue to handicap nursing students even into their senior year (Rachal et al., 2007). Inadequate reading skills and preparation for class (Hendry & Farley, 2006; Igbo et al., 2011; Wolkowitz & Kelly, 2010), poor note-taking skills (Hendry & Farley; Pauk & Owens, 2011), and lack of assignment completion (McGann & Thompson, 2008; Williams, 2010) also contribute to the lack of knowledge.

Academic interventions to improve lack of knowledge include guidance and assistance in preparation for admission testing, regular nursing class attendance, keeping up with assignments, and academic engagement (Pitt et al., 2012; Williams, 2010). Tutoring (Rheinheimer et al., 2010), mentoring (Donahue & Glodstein, 2013; Jeffreys, 2007), supplemental instruction (Harding, 2012), study group attendance (Jeffreys, 2012; Williams), faculty encouragement and support (Shelton, 2003, 2012), and academic integration (Tinto, 1993) have all been found to be helpful in increasing academic success.

Study skills training is foundational to optimizing students' studying and effective knowledge acquisition. It includes skills such as reading improvement methods, time management, note taking, preparing for lecture and discussion, homework completion, keeping up with assignments, critical thinking training, and other skills (Hendry & Farley, 2006; Pauk & Owens, 2011; Rachal et al., 2007). Study skills training, stress management, and caring faculty support are all interventions that have been found to increase academic success (Jeffreys, 2012; Pryjmachuk et al., 2009; Rheinheimer et al., 2010; Shelton, 2003; Williams, 2010; Wilson, Andrews, & Leners, 2006).

Study skills training has been found to prevent attrition, failure in nursing classes, and failure of NCLEX-RN (Condon et al., 2013; Rachal et al., 2007; Thomas & Baker, 2011). Methods used for this training include study skill courses and seminars (Condon et al.; Igbo et al., 2011), textbooks (Pauk & Owens, 2011), and university websites that include academic success guides and study strategies for students.

Some schools have developed specific retention programs that draw on a variety of retention methods to foster students' academic success. The use of combinations of several retention methods makes it difficult to evaluate the efficacy of a specific single intervention (Stingell & Waddell, 2010). Hence, more research is needed to determine the type of assistance necessary to increase the success of at-risk nursing students as a group and as individuals.

## English Language Skills

Language acquisition is another area of concern. Although learning basic interpersonal communication skills in English may take 2 to 3 years, Hansen and Beaver (2012) point out that it takes 5 to 7 years to reach proficiency in the more formal academic language required for college success. They add that the study of medicine or nursing is equivalent to learning an additional language. For this reason, students from diverse cultural, ethnic, socioeconomic, and language backgrounds may experience a disadvantage (Behnke, Gonzales, & Cox, 2010).

Limited English language skills may result in students not adequately understanding the textbooks, class lecture, discussion, or exam questions (Condon & Drew, 1995). Students who struggle in passing these nursing classes because of limited skills would benefit from taking time out to take remedial English classes before starting nursing classes (Condon et al., 2013). Other at-risk nursing students may be able to pass classes with the help of an English tutor; vocabulary study; learning how to break words down into roots, prefixes and suffixes; and the support of competent caring nursing faculty (Condon et al.).

A recent study reported academic success and graduation rates for more than 90 percent of the ethnically diverse at-risk nursing students who enrolled in a pre-clinical preparation program prior to taking clinical nursing classes. This program specifically targeted reading, writing, vocabulary, study skills, and critical thinking (Condon et al., 2013).

Fike et al. (2010) discussed the improvement of educational outcomes for 130 Hispanic students through use of the Keller program. This program broke the content for two courses into modules and then allowed testing and retesting of the modules until competency was achieved. Final exam results showed that the former gap in achievement between Hispanic students and other students had been closed.

Ryan and Dogbey (2012) concluded that international/ESL students need learning environments that foster connectivity. They suggest that this can be fostered by creating classrooms based on caring, respect, authenticity, and small group participation.

# Exam Panic/Anxiety

Underperforming students report greater anxiety and fewer coping mechanisms to deal with their anxiety than students who have greater academic success (English & Gordon, 2004; McGann & Thompson, 2008). Freshmen tend to report greater anxiety than senior students (Rachal et al., 2007). Loss of self-esteem also contributes to exam panic/anxiety (Edwards, Burnhard, Bennett, & Hebden, 2010).

Jeffreys (2012) reports that nursing students with increased exam anxiety often perform poorly on nursing exams. Students with higher levels of anxiety were found to have lower academic achievement and higher attrition rates (Behnke et al., 2010; Fike et al., 2010; Igbo et al., 2011; Pitt et al., 2012; Pryjmachuk et al., 2009). Conversely, thorough preparation, sometimes termed *content mastery*, and practicing good exam skills have been shown to decrease exam anxiety (Thomas & Baker, 2011).

Stress management is an important intervention to decrease exam anxiety (Pauk & Owens, 2011). Studying to understand concepts instead of memorizing details was found to increase self-confidence and decrease anxiety (Thomas & Baker, 2011).

Building a healthy lifestyle, through practices including good eating habits, getting sufficient sleep, exercising, drinking an adequate amount of water, and maintaining a healthy attitude, has been shown to combat exam anxiety (Pauk & Owens, 2011).

# Exam-Taking Skills

Exam-taking skills are often found to be inadequate in underperforming students (English & Gordon, 2004). In preparation for the NCLEX-RN licensure exam, most SONs in the United States use multiple choice question format on nursing exams. This testing format frequently proves to be more taxing than essay format because it moves beyond the mere reproduction of knowledge (Downs, 2012) to applying knowledge correctly in a given scenario. To arrive at the correct answer, the student must effectively reason through several options. Finding the correct answer option demonstrates that a student can apply a new concept correctly (Holtzman, 2008). Test-taking skills can be taught. However, underperforming students have been found to be lacking in many of these skills (English & Gordon).

Interventions to improve strategies around exam taking are available on various university websites (Germanna Community College Tutoring Service, 2007; University of Kansas, n.d.). A summary of TEA exam-taking skills is found in Box 12.3. Problematic test-taking strategies include changing answers, overthinking questions, and misreading questions (Blakeman, 2013; English & Gordon, 2004; Holtzman, 2008; McGann & Thompson, 2008). Rachal et al. (2007) reported that 69 percent of participating senior nursing students improved their test-taking strategies due to involvement in an intervention program despite being in the late stage of their nursing education. Another problem for many students is the lack of knowledge regarding how to apply critical thinking to questions that prioritize nursing interventions in complex nursing situations (English & Gordon; Holtzman; Rachal et al.).

Students who practice writing specific questions related to instructors' lecture notes showed increased performance on multiple choice exams (Hautau et al., 2006). Students who scored higher on vocabulary at the beginning of a semester also scored higher on course exams (Turner & Williams, 2007). Wolkowitz and Kelly (2010) correctly predicted NCLEX-RN pass rates from admission testing scores. Student strategies to reach their

## BOX 12.3

## Summary of Exam Techniques
## for Multiple Choice Questions

A. Be Sure You Know What the Question Is Asking
   - Read question carefully.
   - Underline important words.
   - Try to answer the questions yourself before you look at the answer options.
   - Create a pool of possible answers (jot down key word(s) for each).
B. Consider Each Option Carefully
   - Compare answer options given on exam with your own pool of possible answers.
   - Re-read the question carefully.
   - Read the answer options carefully, underlining key words.
   - Mark each answer option as either true, false, T?, F?, or ?.
C. Use Your Knowledge When Choosing the Best Answer
   - Choose your answer based on what you have learned in the course. Example: Choose answer marked true above one marked ?.
   - Do not choose an answer just because "it sounds good" if you have not heard of it before (in lecture or textbook)—it may be a cleverly worded distractor.
D. Use Your Time Wisely
   - Do not spend too long on any one question.
   - Read the question and answer options carefully (twice if necessary).
   - If you are not sure which choice is correct, guess and mark the question number so you can come back to it if you have time.
   - Do not be in a hurry to leave. Check your paper to be sure you have answered all questions.
   - Check carefully for clerical errors (marking wrong answer by mistake).
   - Read each stem with the answer you have marked to be sure it makes sense.
E. If You Do Not Understand the Question or Answer Option, Ask for Help
   - Ask the instructor to clarify what is not clear.
   - Ask the instructor to "restate" a confusing question or option.
F. Do Not Change Your Answers
   - The only time you should change an answer is when you know why the first answer is wrong and/or why the second answer is right.
   - Never change an answer just because you feel uncertain.

From Loma Linda University School of Nursing, Learning Assistance Program. Copyright 1986, 2006, Loma Linda University.

optimal level should include the development of critical thinking skills with careful study of subject matter (Blackey, 2009).

Poorman and Mastorovich (2008) emphasize the need for exam preparation using critical analysis and metacognitive strategies. To delineate features of underperforming nursing students, DiBartolo and Seldomridge (2005) reviewed 20 years of intervention studies and identified only eight peer-reviewed studies that effectively illustrate positive NCLEX-RN student outcomes via experimental or quasi-experimental outcome studies.

## Other Problems

Problems not addressed by TEA worksheet can be written in under the fifth category of "Other." Math is often cited as a problem area under this category. Math interventions for nursing students include remedial math classes, tutoring in math, referral to the math lab for help, online math instruction and practice, use of nursing math review books, and practice using dosage calculation workbooks (Condon et al., 2013).

Despite the numerous combinations of intervention activities, one critical component that continues to surface is the student need for faculty support, including faculty mentoring (Jeffreys, 2007; McGann & Thompson, 2008; Shelton, 2012; Wilson et al., 2006). There is increasing evidence supporting the need for early faculty interventions (McGann & Thompson). In a landmark study, Shelton (2003) found that perceived faculty support and caring predicted retention and success in a nursing program. Research supports that connecting with caring faculty is a determinant of academic success (Behnke et al., 2010; Igbo et al., 2011; Shelton, 2012; Williams, 2010).

At this point, it is important to note that the general term *faculty support* consists of specific psychologically supportive behaviors (i.e., caring and understanding, encouraging growth, being approachable, demonstrating empathy) and functionally supportive behaviors. For example, faculty need to be available, communicate clearly, give helpful feedback, use fair evaluation methods, assist with problem identification and resolution, and serve as role models (Hansen & Beaver, 2012; Shelton, 2003, 2012). Most nursing education literature concludes that faculty support can significantly affect student success (Evans, 2012; Jeffreys, 2007; Junious, Malecha, Tart, & Young, 2010; Shelton, 2003).

## METHODS

### Design

This study employed a descriptive evaluative design. TEA scores were obtained using TEA worksheets, test scores, test means, and test standard deviations for each exam. Demographic information was obtained from student records.

### Setting

The study was done at a faith-based health sciences university in the western United States. During the spring quarter of 2014, the SON had 54 full-time faculty and 65 contract faculty. The SON programs include 443 generic BS students, 57 AS-BS students, 89 MSN students, 29 certified registered nurse anesthetist (CRNA) students, 25 doctor of nursing practice (DNP) students, and 19 doctor of philosophy (PhD) students, for a total of 662 students.

### Participants

Between October 2007 and May 2010, there were 248 nursing students enrolled at the study site meeting the following inclusion criteria: enrollment in either Fundamentals ($n = 152$) or Med-Surg I ($n = 96$), completion of an initial TEA (either on the first or second

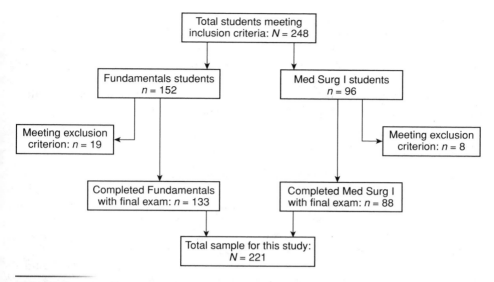

**FIGURE 12.2** Overview of the Participant Inclusion/Exclusion Process.

exam in that course); and scoring below 85 percent (B grade) on that exam. Students were excluded from analysis if they did not take the final exam in the given course the same quarter in which they had their initial TEA. The total number of students excluded was 27 (19 from Fundamentals, 8 from Med-Surg I). The data analysis for this chapter was completed for 221 students (133 from Fundamentals, 88 from Med-Surg I). An overview of the preceding process is provided in Figure 12.2.

# Instruments

TEA worksheet, as described previously, is utilized in this study (see Figure 12.1). The diagnostic procedure utilized for this process includes 10 steps (see Box 12.1). A prescriptive form, Checklist: Suggestions to Improve Exam Performance (see Box 12.2), is given to students to assist in prioritizing specific interventions related to the identified problem areas. The Summary of Exam Techniques for Multiple Choice Questions (see Box 12.3) is given to nursing students during a test-taking seminar and to students participating in TEA.

# Choice of Courses

Fundamentals is a beginning class taken during the first clinical quarter of nursing school. This course is foundational in terms of learning how to process clinically relevant information. Consequently, nursing students go through a major adjustment, as many of them are used to linear thinking and memorization. Now they have to transition to the ability to think critically and apply new concepts to clinical scenarios. Often their previous strategies for test taking do not work because there are not as many direct knowledge questions. TEA helps the students restrategize as they learn to think critically and adjust to this new way of thinking.

The second course chosen for inclusion in this study is the first medical-surgical nursing course, which is taken during the third quarter of the BSN program. Exam questions for this course become increasingly more complex, as students are expected to synthesize their knowledge from the first two quarters of the nursing program and apply critical thinking skills to answer the application questions on course exams.

## Procedures

The University's Institutional Review Board approved the study and evaluation procedures. Participants in the study were identified by a number code.

Students in Fundamentals or Med-Surg I (with an exam score below 85 percent) who requested TEA were scheduled with a LAP facilitator. The facilitators ($n = 14$), many of whom were educators, were all RNs with differing backgrounds and were trained in performing TEA procedure. TEA takes approximately 1 hour.

Exam scores (initial and final) were obtained from Fundamentals and Med-Surg I faculty and were kept secure. Test means and test standard deviations from all test scores for each of the exams in Fundamentals and Med-Surg I were determined using Scantron analysis.

## Data Analysis

Demographic information, admissions testing results, initial exam scores, final exam scores, test means, and test standard deviations were analyzed using paired $t$-tests and chi-square tests using SPSS version 22.0 (SPSS, Inc., 2009).

## RESULTS

A total of 221 nursing students were used in the data analysis (see Figure 12.2). Description of the nursing students in Fundamentals ($n = 133$) and in Med-Surg 1 ($n = 88$) related to age, gender, ethnic background, and prerequisite and cumulative GPA are found in Table 12.1. There were no significant differences in variables between the two groups.

The initial (pre) and final exam (post) scores of students were compared for Fundamentals and Med-Surg I. Standardized scores were used to account for differences in data collected over multiple quarters. There was an improvement of .56 of a standard error unit for Med-Surg I and an improvement of .34 of a standard error unit for Fundamentals (see part A of Table 12.2). The change in mean exam scores was highly significant for both courses ($p = .001, p = < .001$, respectively).

In addition, the change in letter grade from initial score to final score was determined. In Fundamentals, a grade increase of half a letter grade or more was found for 63.2 percent of participants. In Med-Surg I, a grade increase of half a letter grade or more was found for 51.1 percent of participants. Between 19 and 26 percent of students maintained the same level of performance and between 18 and 23 percent did worse in their final exam compared to their initial exam (see part B of Table 12.2).

### TABLE 12.1

## Descriptions of Nurses Who Had Exam Analysis for Fundamentals of Professional Nursing (*n* = 133) or Medical-Surgical Nursing I (*n* = 88)

|  | Fundamentals [%; (*n*)] | Med-Surg I [%; (*n*)] |
|---|---|---|
| Gender |  |  |
| Male | 19.5 (26) | 19.3 (17) |
| Female | 80.5 (107) | 80.7 (71) |
| Ethnicity |  |  |
| Asian | 42.1 (56) | 39.8 (35) |
| Black | 6.0 (8) | 9.1 (8) |
| Caucasian | 25.6 (34) | 27.3 (24) |
| Hispanic | 18.8 (25) | 19.3 (17) |
| Native American | 1.5 (2) | 2.3 (2) |
| Other | 6.0 (8) | 2.3 (2) |
|  | **Mean (SD)** | **Mean (SD)** |
| Age | 23.5 (5.9) | 23.9 (6.3) |
| Prerequisite GPA | 3.3 (0.3) | 3.3 (0.3) |
| Cumulative GPA | 3.5 (2.9) | 3.7 (3.5) |
| Reading | 80.4 (16.7) | 77.3 (17.4) |
| Critical Thinking | 17.6 (3.9) | 16.8 (3.3) |
| Math | 78.3 (13.0) | 75.8 (14.3) |
| Science | 76.9 (11.8) | 79.2 (12.6) |

The change in standardized exam scores (comparing initial with final score) was negatively correlated with the initial standardized exam score ($r = -.57$ for Med-Surg I, $r = -.30$ for Fundamentals). Hence, lower initial exam scores were associated with larger changes in standardized exam scores—that is, changes in standardized scores were most pronounced for students who had lower scores on their first exam (Table 12.3). In Med-Surg I, the changes in standardized exam scores were not correlated with students' pre-admission Critical Thinking, Math, Reading, or Science scores. In Fundamentals, the pre-admission scores in Science, Math, and Critical Thinking were weakly correlated with a change in standardized exam scores. The difference in significance between the two courses is due to size of the correlation coefficients and to the larger sample size for the Fundamentals course (see Table 12.3).

## TABLE 12.2

# Comparison of Changes in Scores and Grades

**A. *Change in Standardized Examination Scores***

| | Initial Exam Mean (SD) | Final Exam Mean (SD) | Change Score Mean (SD) | $p^*$ |
|---|---|---|---|---|
| Fundamentals of Professional Nursing | −.83 (.81) | −.49 (1.04) | −.34 (1.1) | .001 |
| Medical-Surgical Nursing I | −.85 (.84) | −.29 (.88) | −.56 (1.1) | <.001 |

**B. *Change in Letter Grades***

| | Fundamentals ($n=133$) | Med-Surg I ($n=88$) |
|---|---|---|
| Increase by 1/2 letter grade [%; ($n$)] | 63.2 (84) | 51.1 (45) |
| Same grade [%; ($n$)] | 18.8 (25) | 26.1 (23) |
| Less [%; ($n$)] | 18.0 (24) | 22.7 (20) |

*Paired *t*-test.

## TABLE 12.3

# Correlation With Change Scores

| Variables | Fundamentals of Professional Nursing ($n=133$) | | Medical-Surgical Nursing I ($n=88$) | |
|---|---|---|---|---|
| | $r$ | $p$ | $r$ | $p$ |
| Reading | 0.13 | 0.14 | −.11 | 0.33 |
| Critical Thinking | 0.17 | 0.05 | .09 | 0.4 |
| Math | 0.2 | 0.02 | −.04 | 0.72 |
| Science | 0.23 | 0.007 | 0.11 | 0.3 |
| Initial Exam Score | −.30 | 0.001 | −.57 | <.001 |

*Final standardized score—initial standardized score.

# DISCUSSION

Positive and significant change scores were found when comparing the initial (pre-TEA) and the final exam score (post-TEA). This is noteworthy because the initial exam was shorter and covered less material, whereas the final exam integrated material from the entire course. Therefore, it would be logical to expect the final exam to be more difficult. This would argue against the positive change being a random happening. Perhaps taking the initial exam could be compared to climbing a hill and the final exam compared to climbing a mountain.

Visualize a continuum line with "optimally performing students" at one end and "failing students" at the other end. Underperforming students would fall below the optimally performing students to indicate that they could have performed better. These students often benefit from TEA to diagnose problem areas and prescribe focused interventions. Now on this continuum line, visualize a line at 85 percent where the at-risk students fall and where this study is focused. Even though TEA is available to all students who desire to improve, it is recommended (required in some courses) for students with a score of B− (below 85 percent). Jeffreys (2007) agrees that the cut-off score for students at risk of failing nursing begins at B− (85 percent).

As noted in part B of Table 12.2, there is a negative correlation showing that students further below 85 percent showed more progress than those nearer to 85 percent. Even though scores moved significantly, they were still below the class median. The fact remains that the letter grade did move (increased) half a letter grade or more from the initial exam grade (pre-TEA) to the final exam grade (post-TEA) for both students in Fundamentals (63.2 percent) and students in Med-Surg I (51 percent). This is important because for some students, the change of half a letter grade may make the difference between passing or failing a course. In addition, failing a course can mean that a student is forced to drop out of nursing, often with many unfavorable implications such as loss or delay of a desired career, embarrassment about "not passing," additional financial loss/distress, loss/delay of achieving financial independence, and lower retention rate for the SON. The extra costs invested into student retention have to be compared to the lost tuition that results from students dropping out of the program.

The resulting effect of TEA is often carried over to other courses, thus resulting in promoting student retention. Once a student embraces TEA intervention strategies, critical thinking usually results and academic success/retention increases in all courses.

# LIMITATIONS

Limitations of this study include the relatively small sample size obtained from one baccalaureate SON. Therefore, findings might differ based upon a larger group size or in another geographical area.

The inter-rater reliability of TEA was not tested due to the nature of TEA procedure. Having a different LAP facilitator do a second TEA on the same exam with the same student would not be valid or reliable, because the student would remember the questions, answers, and discussion from the first Exam Analysis. Despite the fact that students experienced TEA process with a variety of facilitators, the results of TEA were still significant.

The pairs of exams compared in the study were not of equal length or difficulty, as the final exams were longer and more comprehensive; however, if this difference changed the results of the comparison, it would logically increase, rather than decrease, the significance of the finding. It was not possible to find exams of equal length, comprehensiveness, and difficulty to compare.

The crippling effect of exam anxiety, as described by study participants, is difficult to measure. For example, exam anxiety may influence both the measuring the level of knowledge and the use of exam-taking skills identified by TEA. A recent Exam Analysis strategy, that of identifying the level of anxiety the student experienced prior to and while taking the exam on a scale of 1 to 10, is now providing additional information to assist faculty and students in planning interventions to improve exam performance.

Each Exam Analysis takes approximately 1 hour to complete, and it is advisable to plan a follow-up appointment to clarify the process and discuss student progress. This may seem to be a lot of time. However, if it assists an at-risk student in passing a class or classes and graduating, it is time well spent.

## IMPLICATIONS FOR NURSING EDUCATION AND PRACTICE

- Further investigation and testing of TEA by nursing programs in various locations.
- Train RN facilitators to perform TEA.
- If the school is not able to support RN facilitators to do TEA on a regular basis, individual faculty members or RN volunteers could study the methods used and assist nursing students by volunteering to do TEA.
- Nursing programs should provide workshops and seminars to teach nursing students study strategies, recommended exam-taking skills and exam anxiety-reducing strategies, and provide faculty development workshops on methods for faculty support and cultural competence.
- Nursing faculty development workshops are important in fostering cultural competence and providing faculty with effective methods for faculty support.
- Nursing faculty should make every effort to give caring support and assistance to all students.

## IMPLICATIONS FOR FURTHER STUDY

- Repeat this research with larger sample sizes and in different areas of the country to further evaluate the usefulness of TEA in increasing academic success.
- Study the long-term effect of TEA on subsequent exams, retention, graduation, and NCLEX-RN results.
- Use qualitative research to describe students' feelings about participating in TEA and discuss how TEA impacted their academic success.

- Study student compliance with prescriptive interventions and the effect of compliance on subsequent academic success.
- Survey TEA participants to learn how they think the process could be improved.
- Survey nursing faculty regarding their perception of TEA and its usefulness in improving academic success.
- Study the most frequent problem categories and subcategories identified by TEA and evaluate whether these categories change on subsequent TEAs.
- Study TEA participants' rankings of different interventions for increasing academic success.
- Study the cost of providing and training RN facilitators to do TEA and compare this cost to the cost of losing students due to academic failure.

## CONCLUSION

This study suggests that TEA is an intervention strategy that encourages at-risk students and increases their academic success. TEA provides a tool for nurse educators to provide educational, psychological, and functional support for at-risk students.

## References

August-Brady, M. M. (2005). The effect of a metacognitive intervention on approach to and self-regulation of learning in baccalaureate nursing students. *Journal of Nursing Education, 44*(7), 297–304.

Balduf, M. (2009). Underachievement among college students. *Journal of Advanced Academics, 20*(2), 274–294.

Behnke, A. O., Gonzales, L. M., & Cox, R. B. (2010). Latino students in new arrival states: Factors and services to prevent youth from stopping out. *Hispanic Journal of Behavioral Sciences, 32*(3), 385–409.

Blackey, R. (2009). So many choices, so little time: Strategies for understanding and taking multiple-choice exams in history. *History Teacher 43*(1), 53–66.

Blakeman, J. R. (2013). Never change answers on examinations: Evidence based practice in nursing education? *Journal of Nursing Education, 52*(8), 421–422.

Caputi, L., & Engelman, L. (2008). *Teaching nursing: The art and science* (vol. 4). Glen Ellyn, IL: College of DuPage Press.

Condon, V. M., & Drew, D. E. (1995). Improving examination performance using exam analysis. *Journal of Nursing Education, 34*(6), 254–261.

Condon, V. M., Morgan, C. J., Miller, E. W., Mamier, I., Zimmerman, G. J., & Mazhar, W. (2013). A program to enhance recruitment and retention of disadvantaged and ethnically diverse baccalaureate nursing students. *Journal of Transcultural Nursing, 24*(4), 397–407.

Davidhizar, R., & Shearer, R. (2005). When your student is culturally diverse. *Health Care Manager, 24*(4), 356–363.

DiBartolo, M., & Seldomridge, L. A. (2005). Review of intervention studies to promote NCLEX-RN success of baccalaureate students. *Nurse Educator, 30*(4), 166–171.

Donahue, N., & Glodstein, S. (2013). Mentoring the needs of nontraditional students. *Teaching and Learning in Nursing, 8*(1), 2–3.

Downs, C. (2012). *Strategies for multiple choice exams.* Retrieved May 1, 2013, from University of Illinois, Chicago, OVCSA Academic

Center for Excellence Web site, http://www.uic.edu/depts/ace/hp_test_strategy.shtml

Edwards, D., Burnhard, P., Bennett, K., & Hebden, U. (2010). A longitudinal study of stress and self-esteem in student nurses. *Nurse Education Today, 30*(1), 78–84.

Ellis, S. O. (2006). Nurse entrance test scores: A predictor of success. *Nurse Educator, 31*(6), 259–263.

English, J. B., & Gordon, D. K. (2004). Successful student remediation following repeated failures on the HESI exam. *Nurse Educator, 29*(6), 266–268.

Evans, D. B. (2012). Examining the influence of noncognitive variables on the intention of minority baccalaureate nursing students to complete their program of study. *Journal of Professional Nursing, 29*(3), 148–154.

Fike, D. S., McCall, K. L., Rachel, C. L., Smith, Q. R., & Lockman, P. R. (2010). Improving educational outcomes of Hispanic students in a professional degree program. *Equity and Excellence in Education, 43*(4), 527–538.

Germanna Community College Tutoring Service. (2007). *Test taking strategies for nurses.* Retrieved May 28, 2013, from http://www.germanna.edu/tutor/Handouts/Nursing/Test_Taking_Strategies_for_Nursing.pdf

Harding, M. (2012). Efficacy of supplemental instruction to enhance student success. *Teaching and Learning in Nursing, 7*(1), 27–31.

Hansen, E., & Beaver, S. (2012). Faculty support for ESL nursing students: Action plan for success. *Nursing Education Perspectives, 33*(4), 246–250.

Hautau. B., Turner, H. C., Carroll, E., Jaspers, K., Parker, M., Krohn, K., et al. (2006). Differential daily writing contingencies and performance on major multiple-choice exams. *Journal of Behavioral Education, 15*(4), 256–273.

Hendry, C., & Farley, A. H. (2006). Essential skills for students returning to study. *Nursing Standard, 21*(6), 44–48.

Holtzman, M. (2008). Demystifying application-based multiple-choice questions. *College Teaching, 56*(2), 114–120. Available from http://web.ebscohost.com.ezp.waldenulibrary.org/ehost/delivery?sid=972fa3b4-97b6-4c97

Igbo, I. N., Straker, K. C., Landson, M. J., Symes, L., Bernard, L. F., Hughes, L. A., et al. (2011). An innovative, multidisciplinary strategy to improve retention of nursing students from disadvantaged backgrounds. *Nursing Education Perspectives, 32*(6), 375–379.

Jeffreys, M. R. (2007). Tracking students through program entry, progression, graduation, and licensure: Assessing undergraduate nursing student retention and success. *Nurse Education Today, 27*(5), 406–419.

Jeffreys, M. R. (2012). *Nursing student retention: Understanding the process and making a difference* (2nd ed.). New York, NY: Springer.

Junious, D. L., Malecha, A., Tart, K., & Young, A. (2010). Stress and perceived faculty support among foreign-born baccalaureate nursing students. *Journal of Nursing Education, 49*(5), 261–270.

McGann, E., & Thompson, J. M. (2008). Factors related to academic success in at-risk senior nursing students. *International Journal of Nursing Education Scholarship, 5*(1), 1–15.

Pauk, W., & Owens, R. J. Q. (2011). *How to study in college* (10th ed.). Boston, MA: Wadsworth Cengage Learning.

Pitt, V., Powis, D., Levett-Jones, T., & Hunter, S. (2012). Factors influencing nursing students' academic and clinical performance and attrition: An integrative review. *Nurse Education Today, 32*(8), 903–913.

Poorman, S. G., & Mastorovich, M. L. (2008). Using metacognitive strategies to help students learn in pretest and posttest review. *Nurse Educator, 33*(4), 176–180.

Poorman, S. G., Mastorovich, M. L., & Webb, C. A. (2011). Helping students who struggle academically: Finding the right level of involvement and living with our judgments. *Nursing Education Perspectives, 32*(6), 369–374.

Pryjmachuk, S., Easton, K., & Lockwood, A. (2009). Nurse education: Factors associated with attrition. *Journal of Advanced Nursing, 65*(1), 149–160.

Rachal, K. C., Daigle, S., & Rachal, W. S. (2007). Learning problems reported by college students: Are they using learning strategies?

*Journal of Instructional Psychology, 34*(4), 191–199.

Rheinheimer, D. C., Grace-Odeleye, B., Francois, G. E., & Kusorgbor, C. (2010). Tutoring: A support strategy for at-risk students. *Teaching and Learning Assistance Review, 15*(1), 23–33.

Ryan, J. G., & Dogbey, E. (2012). Seven strategies for international nursing student success: A review of the literature. *Teaching and Learning in Nursing 7*(3), 103–107.

Shelton, E. N. (2003). Faculty support and student retention. *Journal of Nursing Education, 42*(2), 68–76.

Shelton, E. N. (2012). A model of nursing student retention. *International Journal of Nursing Education Scholarship, 9*(1), 1–16.

SPSS, Inc. (2009). *SPSS user's guide for Windows (version 17.0).* Chicago, IL: Author.

Stingell, L. D., & Waddell, G. R. (2010). Modeling retention at a large public university. Can at-risk students be identified early enough to treat? *Research in Higher Education, 51*(54), 546–572.

Thomas, M. H., & Baker, S. S. (2011). NCLEX-RN success evidence-based strategies. *Nurse Educator, 36*(6), 246–249.

Tinto, V. (1993). *Leaving college: Rethinking the causes and cares of student attrition.* Chicago, IL: University of Chicago Press.

Tinto, V. (2006). Research and practice of student retention: What next? *Journal of College Student Retention, 8*(1), 1–19.

Tinto, V. (2012*). Completing college: Rethinking institutional action.* Chicago IL: University of Chicago Press.

Turner, H., & Williams, R. (2007). Vocabulary development and performance on multiple-choice exams in large entry-level courses. *Journal of College Reading and Learning, 37*(2), 64–81.

University of Kansas. (n.d.). *Academic success guides.* Retrieved May 1, 2013, from http://www.achievement.ku.edu/success-guide

Williams, M. G. (2010). Attrition and retention in the nursing major: Understanding persistence in beginning nursing students. *Nursing Education Perspectives, 31*(6), 362–367.

Wilson, V., Andrews, M., & Leners, D. (2006). Mentoring as a strategy for retaining racial and ethnically diverse students in nursing programs. *Journal of Multicultural Nursing & Health, 12*(3), 17–23.

Wolkowitz, A. A., & Kelly, J. A. (2010). Academic predictors of success in a nursing program. *Journal of Nursing Education, 49*(9), 498–503.

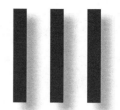

# The NLN Center for Excellence in the Care of Vulnerable Populations

# 13

# The Edmond J. Safra Visiting Nurse Faculty Program:
## An Innovative Model to Enhance Faculty Development and Nursing Education on Parkinson's Disease

**Diane M. Elllis,** MSN, RN, CCRN

**Gwyn M. Vernon,** MSN, CRNP

Parkinson's disease (PD) is a chronic and progressive disorder affecting more than one million individuals and families in the United States, with an associated annual economic burden of more than $34 million (Noyes, Liu, Holloway, & Dick, 2006). PD is the second most common neurodegenerative disorder of adults, with only dementia being more common. One study (Aminoff et al., 2011) found that when hospitalized, patients with PD do not receive their medications on time 75 percent of the time; these are medications that make it possible to move, talk, swallow, walk, feed oneself, and participate in therapy. People with PD are hospitalized 44 percent more than persons without PD, have longer hospital stays, and have higher rates of complications (Aminoff et al.).

Concerned about the nursing care of patients and caregivers, two nurses with expertise in PD noted that it was common for patients to have difficulties when their normal home management routine was altered, as when hospitalization became necessary. Several questions arose: Are nurses taught about PD as undergraduates? Do the patients' difficulties arise from nurses' failure to understand the disease process and the medication regimes required for patients to complete basic activities? Are nursing students mentored on care of patients with PD, and do nurse faculty have the knowledge needed to teach PD content?

## NAMING THE PROBLEM

In 2008, a short survey about PD content was sent to 20 schools of nursing with high *U.S. News & World Report* ratings. These schools were located in large metropolitan areas with supporting academic medical centers and patient access to specialty care.

The survey revealed pertinent information: 70 percent of nurse faculty responsible for PD content did not feel comfortable or confident in their knowledge of the material,

33 percent of the surveyed schools had no PD content in their curricula, and 46 percent of the schools had no clinical mentored experience with patients suffering from PD. A panel of four nurses with expertise in PD reviewed the readings and lecture materials supplied by the schools where PD was taught. More than 97 percent of the materials submitted were rated as out of date, misleading, or irrelevant (Vernon, Bunting-Perry, & Dunlop, 2012).

## THE TRAIN-THE-TRAINER PROGRAM

Survey findings were presented to the Edmond J. Safra Foundation, whose philanthropic portfolio includes several scientific research projects on PD. Funding was obtained to develop the Edmond J. Safra Visiting Nurse Faculty Program to enhance nursing education. The program is based on concepts of the train-the-trainer model. An older educational model, the train-the-trainer model enables experienced personnel to coach and mentor the less experienced using adult theory principles (Duggan, 2013). It was expected that nurse faculty provided with state-of-the-science training in PD content would feel comfortable and confident in educating nursing students.

Goals of the program were established to:

1. Prepare undergraduate nursing students with the knowledge to care for PD patients
2. Enhance the knowledge and skills of nurse faculty to teach students about PD patient care
3. Promote the development of a long-term relationship between nurse faculty and nationwide academic PD centers for future collaboration and to promote scholarly work

The program, now completing its sixth year, brings together nurse faculty and multidisciplinary experts for a 40-contact-hour course consisting of four lectures and workshops in small interactive groups, participation in direct patient care in the clinical arena, attendance at a patient and family support group, and the opportunity to complete an independent project. The immersion course is completed on-site in 4 days. Participants then spend additional time on an independent project of their choosing. The project, mentored by a PD nurse expert where needed, should benefit nursing education or patient care in PD.

Annual surveys are used to evaluate the accomplishment of the program's goals. The surveys request information on the number of students with whom the faculty is involved in teaching about PD; changes to curricula that were made as a result of the faculty's participation in the course; and scholarly work completed during the year of the survey, including collegial relationships with program host faculty.

## MEETING THE PROGRAM GOALS

### Preparing Nursing Students With the Knowledge to Care for Patients

Each year, more than 8,000 nursing students receive up-to-date knowledge about PD as a result of their professors' participation in the program. Nursing students are mentored in the classroom or clinical arena directly by faculty who completed the program; many of these students had no content, outdated content, or very little applicable content on PD prior to their faculty's participation.

Faculty surveys show the implementation of changed content on PD in multiple areas of the curriculum, including medical-surgical nursing, geriatrics, community health, ethics, pharmacology, pathophysiology, and chronic care courses. Faculty report that they seek out clinical exposures for their students and use current information obtained through resources learned in the program. They are creating innovative ways to teach the content, including simulations, evolving case studies, webinars, ethics cases, video cases, and having patients come to the school to assist with the teaching. Some participants have been asked to write questions on PD by companies that provide standardized testing for students.

## Enhancing the Knowledge and Skills of Nurse Faculty

The surveys show all alumni rating their improvement as 100 percent in their ability to teach PD content to nursing students. Comments include "The program was revolutionary in my understanding of PD," "I am empowered to teach about PD," "I am encouraged and anxious to continue my study in PD," and "I had no idea what I did not know about PD."

## Creating a Long-Term Relationship Between Nurse Faculty and PD Center Experts/Fostering Scholarly Work

Scholarly results of the program to date include 20 articles (some are in press), 2 book chapters, and 4 grant-funded research projects. Several faculty provide in-service training on PD outside their school of nursing, such as in nursing homes, assisted living facilities, and home health agencies. A few have started and maintained PD support groups, and one past participant is the resource and training assistant for Canine Partners for Life (Cochranville, PA), serving patients with PD seeking a service dog.

One faculty member is working with her nursing students in Nicaragua to teach community health workers about PD, palliative care measures, and the importance of exercise. Limited medical care exists for patients with PD in larger cities in Nicaragua, and there is little to no available care in rural areas. Another group of scholars is setting up a PD clinic at a nurse-managed faculty practice where telehealth is used to connect the clinic to an academic PD center.

## FUTURE PLANS

The Edmond J. Safra Visiting Nurse Faculty Program is an innovative and interactional faculty development program with team collaboration between nurse faculty and experts at large PD centers. These large, academic, multidisciplinary centers provide expert care for persons with PD and their families. Most have a triad mission of patient care, education, and research. The centers currently involved in the program are listed in Box 13.1.

A goal for the future is to develop a method of more precisely evaluating the program's direct impact on nursing students' knowledge. In the longer term, it is our hope to see the effect of the program on the routine care that patients receive in the hospital, with a decrease in the complication rates experienced by patients with PD.

In addition, it is our hope to continue to develop a cadre of nurse faculty who are knowledgeable and competent in PD care, interested in having an impact on their

---

**BOX 13.1**

## Program Sites to Hosting Parkinson's Disease Centers

Boston University, Boston, MA
Johns Hopkins University, Baltimore, MD
New York University Medical Center, New York, NY
Northwestern University, Chicago, IL
Oregon Health Sciences University, Portland, OR
San Francisco Veterans Medical Center, San Francisco, CA
Struthers Parkinson's Disease Center, Minneapolis, MN
University of Miami, Miami, FL
University of Pennsylvania, Philadelphia, PA

Note: Additional Parkinson's Disease centers are expected to open in 2015. Visit http://www.pdf.org/edmondjsafranursing/ for current information.

---

schools' curricula and student learning, and choose PD as a long-term scholarly interest. This will be done through the gradual expansion of the program into more areas of the United States while fostering the continued development of program participants.

Although elements of the Edmond J. Safra Visiting Nurse Faculty Program are traditional in continuing nursing education, the clinical opportunities that it provides to work directly with patients, families, and support groups make the program unique. Further, the opportunity to embark on an independent project for self-learning provides a stage for continued scholarly interest in this common chronic disorder. This model can easily be adapted to other disease states to improve knowledge and, ultimately, patient care and understanding.

## ACKNOWLEDGMENT

The author would like to express gratitude to Lisette Bunting-Perry, PhD, RN, who cofounded the Edmond J. Safra Visiting Nurse Faculty Program, and to the Edmond J. Safra Foundation for funding the program. Those seeking further information are invited to visit http://www.pdf.org/edmondsjsafranursing/.

---

### References

Aminoff, M. J., Christine, C. W., Friedman, J. H., Chou, K., Lyons, K., Pahwa, R., et al. (2011). Management of the hospitalized patient with Parkinson's disease: Current state of the field and need for guidelines. *Parkinsonism and Related Disorders, 17*(3), 139–145.

Duggan, T. (2013). *What is the train the trainer model?* Retrieved June 19, 2015, from http://work.chron.com/train-trainer-model-5463.html

Noyes, K., Liu, H., Holloway, R., & Dick, A. (2006). Economic burden associated with Parkinson's disease on elderly Medicare beneficiaries. *Movement Disorders, 21*(3), 362–372.

Vernon, G. M., Bunting-Perry, L., & Dunlop, R. (2012). Edmond J. Safra Visiting Nurse Faculty Program: An innovative strategy to advance Parkinson's disease patient care [Abstract]. *Movement Disorders, 27*(Suppl. 1), 942.

# 14

# MEDTAPP Mentor:
# Improving Health Care
# for Medicaid Clients

**Pamela K. Rutar,** EdD, MSN, RN, CNE
**Lori Arietta,** MSN/Ed, RN

Caring for clients enrolled in Medicaid and other forms of medical assistance can be a challenge, causing a shortage of healthcare providers to service this population; however, an increase in trained quality providers may help to alleviate some of these challenges. Disparities in care among patients with low socioeconomic status persist and can negatively affect patient outcomes (Bernheim, Ross, Krumholz, & Bradley, 2008). This chapter describes a program aimed at "supporting the development and retention of additional healthcare practitioners with skills and competencies to serve the Medicaid population using emerging healthcare delivery models and evidence-based practices, such as health homes and integrated behavioral and physical health service delivery" (Medicaid Technical Assistance and Policy Program Healthcare Access Initiative, 2012, p. 1).

The program uses an interprofessional model to address knowledge gaps and a mentor model to provide field experience in caring for those enrolled in Medicaid. This chapter describes the pilot project implemented with nursing and social work students. An evaluation of the project based on student and mentor responses to a postprogram survey is provided.

## PLANNING THE CURRICULUM

The Institute of Medicine (2011) has called for changes in the education of nurses. Recommendations include the following key message:

- Nurses should be full partners with medicine and other health professions in the redesign of health care (p. S-6).

Additionally, the Quality and Safety Education for Nurses (QSEN) initiative identified teamwork and collaboration as one of its six core competencies (Cronenwett et al., 2007). Each of these recognizes the importance of interprofessional teamwork, communication, and collaboration as important factors in the delivery of high-quality, safe, and effective health care.

The mentoring program of the Medicaid Technical Assistance and Policy Program (MEDTAPP) was developed through the Healthcare Access Initiative to address issues of provider preparation and education as it relates to the health care of the medically underserved and those on Medicaid assistance. The project was partially funded by the MEDTAPP Healthcare Access Initiative. Program goals included the following:

1. Increase the number of new practitioners into healthcare positions primarily serving the Medicaid population in the areas of nursing and social work by June 2013.

2. Establish an interdisciplinary mentoring project to perpetuate the education and training of healthcare professionals in serving the Medicaid population.

3. Perpetuate the project through participation of graduates to act as mentors for future students by the end of June 2013.

The pilot group included student nurses and student social workers in the final semester of preparation before graduation. The program employed two strategies for educating students. The first was a monthly interprofessional seminar presentation of topics related to caring for the Medicaid population. The second was a clinical component in which students were paired with same-discipline professionals working at sites that serve the population. The oversight team for the project included nursing and social work faculty at a growing urban university in the Midwest. All members of the oversight team worked together to develop content to complement that which students previously learned as part of their respective preparatory programs.

## SEMINAR SESSIONS

The seminar sessions were designed as an interprofessional experience for the students, which has been shown to provide students with valuable insights and knowledge that are useful when they enter the workplace (Chan, Mok, Po-Ying, & Man-Chun, 2009; Dunfrene, 2012). The sessions provided students with a combined learning experience where topics related to care of the Medicaid population could be explored. Both nursing and social work students received introductory content on many of the topics in their respective preparatory program. These seminar sessions were designed to address these previously learned topics in more depth. Speakers for each topic were selected from local public health and social service agencies. Topics covered in the sessions included:

- Description of Current Medicaid Programs and Qualifications for Enrollment in Each Program
- The Affordable Care Act and the Projected Impact on Care for the Underserved
- Quality Improvement Processes
- Issues of Culture in Caring for the Medicaid Population
- Advocacy for the Medicaid Client

The content was selected and sequenced so that important concepts could be integrated into the clinical area. Speakers shared best practices and experiences related to their topics.

After the presentation by the speakers, students engaged in discussions of case studies related to the content. The ensuing discussions offered students insight into the roles of the other discipline, as well as ideas about how to work together for the benefit of the patient.

## CLINICAL COMPONENT

A mentoring model was chosen for the clinical component, as mentors have been demonstrated to support successful transition into the workplace (Cottingham, DiBartolo, Battistoni, & Brown, 2011; Fox, 2011). Mentors were selected from the available preceptors used by the School of Nursing and the Department of Social Work for a capstone course. Mentors were expected to meet discipline-specific experiential preceptor requirements in addition to experience working with the Medicaid population.

Mentees were selected from lists of students after completion of an interest form. Some students opted out of the program, but a total of 23 social work and 20 nursing students completed the program. Students signed an agreement to comply with the requirements of the project, which included:

1. Complete this project in the last semester of the preparatory program.
2. Meet the precepted experience requirements for their discipline.
3. Seek employment with a provider of Medicaid services.
4. Attend seminar sessions and complete records as requested by the program.

Clinical sites included a variety of community and hospital-based settings providing care to Medicaid clients in pediatrics, mental health, adolescent mental health, and adult health. The clinical sites enabled students to develop knowledge, skills, and attitudes related to the QSEN competencies, including patient-centered care, teamwork and collaboration, evidence-based practice, quality improvement, safety, and informatics within the context of caring for Medicaid clients (Cronenwett et al., 2007). An example of one such application is a nursing student who was caring for a school-age child who was newly diagnosed with diabetes mellitus. The child's family was planning a move to another state, and the student was concerned about the knowledge deficit and a possible lack of resources for the child after the move. With the cooperation of the mentor and with suggestions by social workers during the discussion, the student nurse crafted a transition plan for the child. Such experiences reinforce concepts covered in the educational sessions.

## PROGRAM EVALUATION

An online evaluation survey was administered to participants in the month after the program. Both mentors and mentees reported that the program was beneficial in aiding their understanding of how to address the needs of the Medicaid population. Because the program was a pilot, there were recommendations for changes, such as providing a more thorough orientation for mentors and mentees and exploring topics in further depth. Mentor participation in the sessions was limited due to conflicting work schedules, but most recommendations included continuing the seminar sessions on Saturdays as scheduled. The program was successful in meeting initial objectives; nearly 100 percent of participants stated that they were seeking employment with a Medicaid provider.

# CONCLUSION

An interprofessional curriculum aimed at meeting the needs of the Medicaid population achieved the first two program objectives, with all but one student obtaining employment with a provider of services to Medicaid clients. The second objective (to perpetuate the program) is pending; many of the graduates expressed an interest in serving as mentors once they gain the necessary experience.

Future plans for the program include the addition of students from other healthcare disciplines, such as medicine and physical therapy, for the purpose of recruiting additional providers to service the population of interest.

Additionally, work will begin to address continuation of the program beyond the terms of the grant funding. The program works well with the existing curriculum and could be offered as an interprofessional value-added component for students. Through this program, the deployment of a healthcare work force attuned to the needs of the Medicaid population is possible now and in the future.

## References

Bernheim, S. M., Ross, J. S., Krumholz, H. M., & Bradley, E. H. (2008). Influence of patients' socioeconomic status on clinical management decisions: A qualitative study. *Annals of Family Medicine, 6*(1), 53–59.

Chan, E. A., Mok, E., Po-Ying, A. H., & Man-Chun, J. H. (2009). The use of interdisciplinary seminars for the development of caring dispositions in nursing and social work students. *Journal of Advanced Nursing, 65*(12), 2658–2667.

Cottingham, S., DiBartolo, M. C., Battistoni, S., & Brown, T. (2011). Partners in nursing: A mentoring initiative to enhance nurse retention. *Nursing Education Perspectives, 32*(4), 250–255.

Cronenwett, L., Sherwood, G., Barnsteiner, J., Disch, J., Johnson, J., Mitchell, P., et al. (2007). Quality and safety education for nurses. *Nursing Outlook, 55*(3), 122–131.

Dunfrene, C. (2012). Health care partnerships: A literature review of interdisciplinary education. *Journal of Nursing Education, 51*(4), 212–216.

Fox, K. C. (2011). Mentor program boosts new nurses' satisfaction and lowers turnover rate. *Journal of Continuing Education in Nursing, 41*(7), 311–316.

Institute of Medicine. (2011). *The future of nursing: Leading change, advancing health.* Washington, DC: National Academies Press.

Medicaid Technical Assistance and Policy Program Healthcare Access Initiative, Ohio Colleges of Medicine Government Resource Center. (2012). *Current project continuation and expansion guidance.* Columbus, OH: Ohio Colleges of Medicine Government Resource Center.

# IV

# The NLN Center for Transformational Leadership

# 15

# Inspiring Future Faculty:
## Innovative Clinical Experiences to Encourage Faculty Development in Nursing Students

**Carol Lynn Maxwell-Thompson,** MSN, RN, FNP-C
**Sarah W. Craig,** PhD, MSN, RN, CCNS, CCRN, CSC
**Kelly Riley,** BSN, RN
**Emily Drake,** PhD, RN, FAAN

There is a growing nursing shortage in the United States; underpinning the nursing shortage is a significant nursing faculty shortage (National League for Nursing, 2013). The American Association of Colleges of Nursing (AACN) reported that in 2011, U.S. nursing schools denied enrollment to 75,587 qualified nursing applicants for BSN and graduate nursing programs; two-thirds of the nursing schools surveyed cited faculty shortages as the main reason for not accepting all qualified nursing applicants (AACN, 2012a).

This chapter describes an innovative approach involving nursing students (both RN-to-BSN and senior-level pre-licensure students) in clinical teaching experiences that are designed to achieve clinical learning goals, inspire future nursing faculty, and reduce the nursing shortage gap, both in practice and in academia.

## PRACTICUM IN CLINICAL TEACHING

Innovative experiences in clinical education were developed as an option for post-licensure students (RN-to-BSN) and as an elective course offering for senior-level pre-licensure students (BSN and direct-entry clinical nurse leader [CNL] students). Since 2010, more than 30 students have participated in these experiences. Program evaluation has been positive. This practicum has a potential three-pronged benefit:

1. Advanced students are provided the opportunity to explore faculty teaching and clinical instruction as a potential career path,

2. Younger students have increased support and guidance during their clinical experiences, and

3. Clinical instructors gain valuable assistance mentoring students on the clinical unit.

## Post-Licensure Students

Post-licensure RN-to-BSN students typically participate as assistant clinical instructors (ACIs) in areas where they have some work experience. These RN-to-BSN students are able to teach undergraduate students under the guidance of experienced faculty. The RN-BSN students are oriented to the role by working alongside the clinical faculty and can be assigned to lead a small group of four to five students during the clinical day. The ACIs are responsible for coaching their group in:

- Identifying issues and creating a plan of care
- Collaborating with other members of the healthcare team
- Performing and documenting physical assessments
- Implementing and evaluating nursing care, communication, and problem solving

Because RN-to-BSN students are licensed, they are able to assist in supervising medication administration. The ACIs also provide feedback during postconference and review clinical preparation worksheets and clinical assignments to gain experience with grading and evaluation.

RN-to-BSN students typically enter the program with many years of experience in a variety of settings. They are confident, mature practitioners. Many of these RN students have served as preceptors for new graduates and new employees, and may even have some experience with clinical teaching. These students are practicing RNs with a wealth of clinical experience. This practicum reflects and engages their experiences and helps to meet their need for higher-level clinical experiences (AACN, 2012b).

## Pre-Licensure Students

Another elective clinical leadership course and clinical teaching practicum is offered to advanced senior undergraduate BSN and pre-licensure CNL students. Despite the CNL student already possessing a baccalaureate degree, these two groups may share a lack of nursing experience. This practicum builds on peer mentoring and skill development.

To be chosen for this experience, these students secure the agreement and recommendation of a clinical faculty member who worked with them previously in the hospital setting. These pre-licensure assistant clinical instructors (p-ACIs) work closely with the clinical faculty member. Prior to every clinical experience, the ACIs meet with the faculty to specifically plan responsibilities, debrief, and plan for future clinical experiences. The p-ACIs are able to supervise most aspects of patient care, although medication administration and sterile procedures are still performed under the supervision of clinical faculty.

All students who participate in the clinical teaching elective meet for a weekly classroom discussion. These sessions are focused on debriefing the clinical teaching experiences, as well as discussing current nursing issues and educational methods. The ACIs are additionally responsible for writing weekly logs about their teaching experiences and researching current literature on nursing education.

## EVALUATION

The teaching practicum culminates in the following evaluations of the experience:

1. Feedback from students
2. Feedback from both groups of ACIs
3. Feedback from faculty

A summary of these evaluations follows.

## Feedback from Students

The undergraduate students reported increased confidence under the guidance of an ACI. They reported learning critical time management, organizational techniques, and priority setting from the ACI. They stated that they developed enhanced communication skills with patients, families, staff, and faculty.

ACIs demonstrated how to enter a room and engage a new patient, and they served as strong role models. These peer-mentor relationships often continued outside of the clinical experience. For example, one young struggling nursing student was coached and mentored by a senior student and was able to be successful in continuing her nursing education. This kind of effort to promote student success and retention can be quite valuable.

One disadvantage was that some of the students became heavily dependent on the ACIs and found it difficult to act without their guidance. Conversely, some of the more independent students did not value the insight and input of ACIs. This may have been due to the nature of the peer relationship.

Undergraduate students generally appreciated the opportunity to learn from more experienced colleagues. Written comments at the end of the semester reflected a common theme:

- "I think that having clinical assistants for our first clinical was very useful because they knew exactly what we were going through."
- "I felt like they were really approachable because they were in the same place as us so recently, and they never passed any judgment because they knew exactly how we felt."
- "They made my clinical experience far more enjoyable. As a result, I felt more confident."

## Feedback from Both Groups of Assistant Clinical Instructors

Students who served as ACIs reported several motivations to participate:

- Leadership development
- Commitment to nursing

- "Looks good on my resume"
- Provides great discussion points during job interviews

They also shared that the course provides a real opportunity to explore faculty teaching and clinical instruction as a potential career path. For example, one RN-to-BSN ACI now teaches a clinical group for a local community college on the same unit where she taught in this clinical elective. By enrolling in this elective, she earned academic credit and clinical teaching experience, and she was oriented to the unit, staff, and clinical teaching role.

On the clinical unit, the ACIs were also able to refine and validate their own knowledge and skills as they engaged with students. They were motivated to teach and apply the latest evidence-based practice. They learned to assess individual students, adapt teaching strategies for different learning styles, and identify crucial teachable moments. Finally, by participating in the weekly, midterm, and final evaluation process, they practiced providing constructive feedback to students.

ACI students also reported that nonclinical activities included learning about course management. They were involved in planning prior to the start of the clinical rotations. They helped to develop the course website, create new clinical teaching tools, and evaluate the effectiveness of current teaching tools and methods. As a result, they gained a broader perspective of the educator role, including the time and effort necessary to design meaningful learning experiences.

Many senior students (p-ACIs) found this elective particularly helpful in preparing for the NCLEX-RN®. Through teaching, these students solidified their knowledge about disease processes and pharmacology. Many clinical assistants expressed the feeling that "you don't know what you know until you have to teach it."

## Feedback from Faculty

Having an ACI on the unit reduced strain on the faculty and clinical staff during the clinical day. While the ACI worked with students on basic vital signs, assessments, blood glucose monitoring, incision care, and computer documentation, the faculty member was free to assist with higher-level tasks such as medication administration and sterile procedures.

However, working with an ACI takes time and effort. It also requires good organizational skills and frequent communication between the faculty and the assistants. Orienting and coaching the ACI is time consuming and labor intensive at the beginning of the process; however, across the semester, the faculty demands reduced significantly. Overall, faculty reported that this experience was very rewarding as they helped to develop the next generation of nursing faculty.

## IMPLEMENTATION, RECOMMENDATIONS, AND CONCLUSION

Faculty considering implementation of this process might want to begin with a pilot course prior to full implementation. Awarding faculty release time to work on course development provides time for faculty to focus on challenges to implementation at their school, and ensures faculty commitment before launching into a larger program. Selecting one student volunteer as an ACI for part of a semester or for a full semester as an independent study may allow for faculty to learn about the scope of the work involved. Thoughtful and deliberate planning is needed to ensure that this experience is truly beneficial for all parties—students, faculty, and clinical staff.

The clinical electives reported in this chapter can serve as a model for other schools of nursing. They were designed with the intention of inspiring future nursing faculty while also providing an enhanced clinical experience for novice nursing students with the additional outcome of reducing demands on clinical faculty time yielding more oversight of, and a better experience for, clinical students. This is an innovative option that schools of nursing can consider to help meet the demands of the current faculty shortage.

## References

American Association of Colleges of Nursing. (2012a). *Nursing faculty shortage fact sheet.* Retrieved June 19, 2015, from http://www.aacn.nche.edu/media-relations/Faculty-ShortageFS.pdf

American Association of Colleges of Nursing. (2012b). *White paper: Expectations for practice experiences in the RN to baccalaureate curriculum.* Retrieved June 19, 2015, from http://www.aacn.nche.edu/aacn-publications/white-papers/RN-BSN-White-Paper.pdf

National League for Nursing. (2013). *Nursing faculty shortage fact sheet.* Retrieved June 19, 2015, from http://www.nln.org/docs/default-source/advocacy-public-policy/nurse-faculty-shortage-fact-sheet-pdf.pdf?sfvrsn=0

# 16

# Art of Nursing:
# The Guiding Principles of an Innovative IPE Teaching-Learning Initiative

**Jeanne M. Walter,** PhD, RN, FAAMA
**Sara Wilson-McKay,** PhD
**Carley G. Lovell,** MA, MS, RN, WHNP-BC
**Jesse S. White,** BFA, MAE
**Meredith Hertel,** BA, MAE
**Susan L. Lindner,** MSN, RNC-OB

The American Association of Colleges of Nursing (2008) and the Institute of Medicine (IOM, 2010) of the National Academies outline the development of astute observation and clinical reasoning skills as essential to nursing education programs. These entities identify integrative liberal education strategies to achieve this end. Clinical reasoning influences what nurses notice and how they interpret findings, respond, and reflect on their responses. This is vital to improved patient outcomes (IOM). Standard approaches to teaching these skills include lectures and practice in a clinical setting; however, there is a need for an innovative, comprehensive curriculum (Pellico, Friedlaender, & Fennie, 2009) that challenges students to move beyond surface assessment and increases their capacity for thoughtful, productive action in the workplace. Responding to this need, our research team developed Art of Nursing, a novel, art-based teaching-learning initiative that brings together art education graduate students, beginning nursing students, and clinical faculty. This rich interprofessional relationship is pivotal in our quest to enhance clinical reasoning at the bedside.

## BACKGROUND

A number of research initiatives present art-based learning as a successful means of introducing depth to traditional clinical study (Bardes, Gillers, & Herman, 2001; Pellico et al., 2009; Wikström, 2000). Investigations into the benefits of merging these two disciplines focus on enhancing students' abilities to engage in complex observation (Pellico et al.).

Shapiro, Rucker, and Beck (2006) label this process "deep seeing" and describe how art observation and analysis teaches students to consider detail, reflect on and revisit first impressions, and determine significance. Research confirms that after engaging with artworks, students generate a greater number of sophisticated observations (Bardes et al.; Naghshineh et al., 2008) and extract more meaning from those observations (Inskeep & Lisko, 2001). Students may also think about how they arrive at conclusions, not simply about the conclusions themselves, preparing them to deal with multilayered problems that often involve ambiguous information (Herman, 2011).

## SIGNIFICANCE

Art of Nursing emphasizes interprofessional education (IPE) through dialogic iterative cycles of development and locates those processes in meaningful art environments to foster a humanistic approach to health care. Our program employs action research design to access and analyze "illuminative experiences" that might otherwise go unconsidered (Stringer, 2004).

Our interprofessional partnership generates new connections between art and nursing to provide participants with robust opportunities for professional growth, thereby enriching study and practice in both fields.

Although our research team is not alone in investigating art as a means for reimagining clinical education, we focus on our guiding principles (discussed later) to nurture the emergence of new knowledge through more than one avenue of inquiry. We emphasize a process of thinking about thinking, referred to as metacognitive awareness (Flavell, 1978), as a firm foundation for beginning nursing students to examine their interactions and communications with patients, families, and colleagues in the clinical setting. Nursing students leave each art experience with enhanced skills in perception, communication, and reflection, gaining fresh insight into the complexities of the nursing profession.

## THEORETICAL/CONCEPTUAL BASIS

Art of Nursing gives students time to refine metacognitive awareness by effectively linking the "knowing and doing" of education (Brown, Collins, & Duguid, 1989). Solidified through written reflection, moments of situated learning (Brown et al.; Lave & Wenger, 1990) occur when participants examine the structures of individual and collective thought; how and why those structures change; why it is important to be cognizant of those shifts; and moreover, how thinking affects clinical care. The museum provides a critical backdrop for this learning. By pulling environment into teaching, art educators challenge students to consider circumstance, organization, and materiality within their observations.

## THE ART OF NURSING MUSEUM EXPERIENCE

The Art of Nursing program is implemented with our pre-licensure nursing students in their first clinical-based course (Technologies of Nursing Practice). Our students consist of two cohorts: traditional baccalaureate and accelerated baccalaureate (second degree

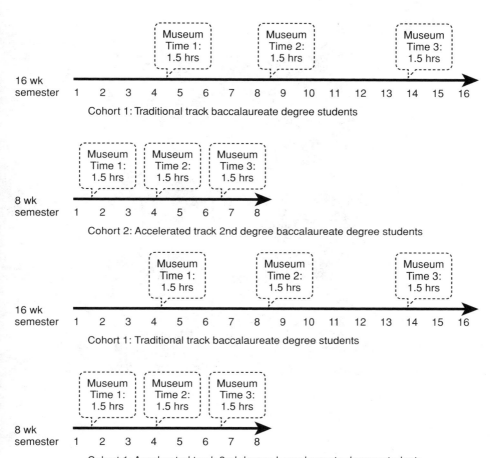

**FIGURE 16.1** Art of Nursing Intervention Schema.

students). Students participate in the Art of Nursing museum experience three times during a 16- and 8-week semester, respectively, at the museum (Figure 16.1).

The Museum of Fine Arts is a state-supported, privately endowed educational institution created for the benefit of the citizens of this urban community. Following a morning in their clinical rotation at the medical center, each student group (consisting of 10 students) and their clinical instructor meet with the art educator student facilitator at the museum in the afternoon (generally 2:30 PM to 4:00 PM). Art education students have preselected artworks (e.g., paintings, sculptures) that are chosen for their unique features and ability to generate thoughtful consideration and communication. The art education students design a set of perception and communication activities related to the artworks. Each group then views and discusses specific artworks—usually three per museum session. For example, using the painting *Heartbreak* (Pearce, 1884) by Charles Sprague-Pearce (Figure 16.2) as the focus, the art education student may lead a discussion of the group by asking the following sample questions and/or implementing activities:

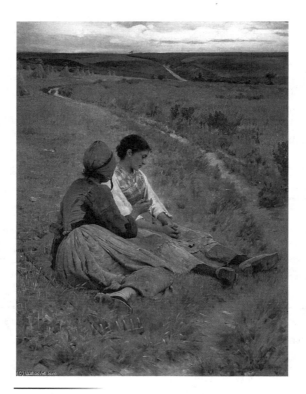

**FIGURE 16.2** Charles Sprague-Pearce, *Heartbreak* [painting] 61.62 in. × 47.37 in., 1884, Museum of Fine Arts.

- What's going on in this painting? What relationships do you see? Point to specific details that can be observed.
- Build a narrative or story about the artwork in smaller groups (three to four students). Come back to the larger group to share the different narratives that you generated.
- How did each group approach the narrative-building process? What are the similarities and differences between the narratives? What might have contributed to these?
- What specific details led you to build that narrative?
- Has your view of the piece changed after hearing opinions and ideas of your peers?

The clinical instructor may suggest or ask students how a particular observation or interpretation may relate to the clinical environment or patient care. Students frequently are able to make powerful connections with their clinical experiences or professional practice. The choice of specific artworks and pedagogical strategies may vary depending on previous museum experiences and student reflections. Following each museum experience,

## BOX 16.1

### Sample Prompt and Nursing Student Reflections

*Prompt:* How has the Art of Nursing program affected your teaching methods and development as a facilitator of this IPE initiative?

*Art Student Reflections:*

- "The Art of Nursing program has allowed me to become a more effective art educator through encouraging the development of my ability to question, respond, and adapt in a thoughtful and reflective manner. These sessions have pushed me to consider various audiences and applications of the arts, helping me to understand the ways that art can facilitate emotional and cognitive growth across disciplines and backgrounds. I also have learned to build an educational space that relies heavily on dialogue and exchange—allowing myself and participants the flexibility to explore how we understand, communicate, and reflect together. These skills easily transfer to my practice in the classroom."

- "I am now more adept at structuring meaningful conversations as well as responding authentically to my students. In this way, I achieve a classroom environment where students feel comfortable engaging with unfamiliar ideas and investigating new ways of thinking. Additionally, because of the way the Art of Nursing program is designed, I have learned to reflect honestly about my experiences and to change my approach when something does not work. This capacity to adapt is crucial to maintaining an active teaching and learning environment, and I am lucky to have had the opportunity to hone these skills in such an exciting educational experience."

NOTE: Art student educators reflect on the meaning of each Art of Nursing experience. These excerpts are used with permission from the reflection log of Hertel (2014).

art education students give a single prompt (Box 16.1) to nursing students relative to the experience. Nursing students then write a brief time-designated reflection of their experience. We qualitatively analyzed these responses (more than 500 to date) and have identified three categorical themes:

1. Reflection
2. Perception
3. Communication

Art education students also reflect on their experiences facilitating each learning initiative (Box 16.2). The experience provides the opportunity to expand their viewpoints and repertoire of teaching techniques through enhanced interactions and communications with nursing students and faculty.

## PROGRAMMATIC GUIDING PRINCIPLES

Three principles position Art of Nursing at the forefront of developing research.

---

## BOX 16.2

### Sample Prompt and Art Education Student Reflections

*Prompt:* How did your critical engagement with works of art today connect to your development as a nurse?

*Nursing Student Reflections:*

- "Communication techniques were a key element of discussion. Some students described the scene using concrete details, while others told a story about the picture first. This generated a discussion about handoff of a patient and that none of the 'other things' matter without providing the story of the patient. There was also conversation surrounding presenting the general meaning first versus presenting the details of the picture first...and which method was more useful to the drawer. We related this to SBAR report technique and that we start with the general typically and move to more specific content (Situation, Background, Assessment, and Recommendation). We also talked about how nurses give verbal report and then do a brief report at the bedside."

- "I had not thought about this too much before since we focus mainly on our own personal observations of patients but now I consider the power of a second opinion. If two people can work together to get a more thorough observation on a patient that could increase their chance of getting healthy then it would be helpful to increase collaboration within the healthcare setting."

NOTE: Nursing students respond to query in Bb© Discussion Board. From Walter (2013). *Technologies of Nursing Practice.* Virginia Commonwealth University. Blackboard Inc©. E-Learning Platform: http://blackboard.vcu.edu

## Interprofessional Collaboration

IPE is defined as "students from two or more professions learn[ing] about, from and with each other to enable effective collaboration and improve health outcomes" (World Health Organization, 2010). By linking the two seemingly disparate fields of art and nursing, we embrace "outsideness" as a catalyst for deeper understanding (Bakhtin, 1986), using art to reveal less frequently explored characteristics of clinical practice, and vice versa (Hsu, 2010). We engage across disciplines to move beyond the limitations of our own expertise and expand our capacity for reflective practice.

The literature describes IPE programs that focus almost exclusively on the clinical-medical field, providing little evidence that frameworks have been extended to incorporate other professions. In our model, art educators are integral to the IPE relationship. The guiding principle of interprofessional collaboration assures integrity in our program design so that both art educators and nurses benefit professionally, demonstrating the benefits of interdisciplinary education across art and science.

## Instructional Focus on Dialogic Looking

Art of Nursing's participatory small group setting (1 art educator and 1 clinical instructor to 10 students) sparks interprofessional growth in students by increasing their capacity for clear verbal exchange and sensitive engagement with colleagues and patients. Through shared discussion, students use visual details as building blocks for further assessment to strengthen their understanding of *how* and *why* they arrive at conclusions (Wilson McKay & Monteverde, 2003). This collaborative processing situates individual knowledge in unfamiliar contexts to create new meaning (Bakhtin, 1986) and challenges students to reach outside the "proverbial box of their conventional thinking" (Hsu, 2010, p. 211) to gain critical awareness of their role as a nursing professional.

## Evaluation and Revision

Although we reference key clinical learning standards in the design of our curriculum, responsive development remains at the core of our practice. This attention to critical praxis reflects our commitment to authentic transformation (Freire, 1970). Questioning the underlying beliefs and assumptions that pervade traditional definitions of clinical education supports active, meaningful learning (Sandars, Singh, & McPherson, 2012).

Our ongoing focus on evaluation and revision includes collaborative planning based on session assessment, participants' written reflections, staff reflection following each session, and review of research data. The value that we place on this principle ensures a responsive program, resisting prescriptive curriculum that may inhibit learner engagement.

## FUTURE DIRECTIONS

Art of Nursing situates participatory, interprofessional dialogue in an architecture of critical reflection and iterative development. Our innovative program model captures the tension between firm learning standards and open-ended inquiry, using that dynamic to produce experiences that are highly relevant to our students' development of clinical reasoning.

IPE is widely acknowledged as critical to the instruction of all healthcare profes-sionals (Charles, Barring, & Lake, 2011), but research-based assessment of IPE models and programmatic outcomes is limited. Art of Nursing is significant because it focuses not only on the design of an IPE model but also establishes specific, measureable aims and outcomes that address methodological challenges in implementation and evaluation. Although this early work has focused on the qualitative aspects of our model, we are expanding our research to incorporate mixed methods to better assess and quantify pro-gram effectiveness. We will be assessing metacognition in our future student cohorts. Metacognition refers to the ability to reflect upon, understand, monitor, and control one's learning (Martinez, 2006; Schraw & Dennison, 1994). To this end, we will employ Schrawe and Dennison's Metacognitive Awareness Scale (MAS) to measure how students "think about their thinking" prior to the Art of Nursing experience and how it changes over time. We anticipate that findings from the MAS, combined with our qualitative data, will provide a more robust depiction of the Art of Nursing IPE initiative and add further clarity to ongoing development of our pedagogical model.

## References

American Association of Colleges of Nursing. (2008). *The essentials of baccalaureate education for professional nursing practice.* Retrieved June 19, 2015, from http://www.aacn.nche.edu/education-resources/baccessentials08.pdf

Bakhtin, M. (1986). *Speech genres and other late essays.* Austin, TX: University of Texas Press.

Bardes, C., Gillers, D., & Herman, A. (2001). Learning to look: Developing clinical observational skills at an art museum. *Medical Education, 35*(12), 1157–1161.

Brown, J. S., Collins, A., & Duguid, S. (1989). Situated cognition and the culture of learning. *Educational Researcher, 18*(1), 32–42. Available from http://www.jstor.org/stable/1176008

Charles, G., Barring, V., & Lake, S. (2011). What's in it for us? Making the case for interprofessional field education experiences for social work students. *Journal of Teaching in Social Work, 31*(5), 579–593.

Flavell, J. H. (1978). Metacognitive development. In J. M. Scandura & C. J. Brainerd (Eds.), *Structural/process models of complex human behavior* (pp. 213–245). Alphen aan den Rijn, The Netherlands: Sijthoff & Noordhoff.

Freire, P. (1970). *Pedagogy of the oppressed.* New York: Continuum Publishing.

Herman, A. (2011). The art of perception: Museums breaking ground in law enforcement programs. *Journal of Museum Education, 36*(1), 81–89.

Hertel, M. (2014). Art of Nursing art educator reflection log. Unpublished.

Hsu, P. (2010). Beyond space and across time: Non-finalized dialogue about science and religion discourse. *Cultural Studies of Science Education, 5*(1), 201–212.

Inskeep, S. J., & Lisko, S. A. (2001). Alternative clinical nursing experience in an art gallery. *Nurse Educator, 26*(3), 117–119.

Institute of Medicine. (2010). *The future of nursing: Leading change, advancing health.* Retrieved June 19, 2015, from http://www.iom.edu/Reports/2010/The-Future-of-Nursing-Leading-Change-Advancing-Health.aspx

Lave, J., & Wenger, E. (1990). *Situated learning: Legitimate peripheral participation.* Cambridge, UK: Cambridge University Press.

Martinez, M. (2006). What is metacognition? *Phi Delta Kappan, 87*(9), 696–699.

Naghshineh, S., Hafler, J. P., Miller, A. R., Blanco, M. A., Lipsitz, S. R., Dubroff, R. P., et al. (2008). Formal art observation training improves medical students' visual diagnostic skills. *Journal of General Internal Medicine, 23*(7), 991–997.

Pellico, L., Friedlaender, L., & Fennie, K. (2009). Looking is not seeing: Using art to improve observational skills. *Journal of Nursing Education, 48*(11), 648–653.

Pearce, C. S. (1884). Heartbreak [painting]. Retrieved June 19, 2015, from http://www.the-athenaeum.org/art/full.php?ID=47480

Sandars, J., Singh, G., & McPherson, M. (2012). Are we missing the potential of action research for transformative change in medical education? *Education for Primary Care, 23*(4), 239. Available from http://leeds.academia.edu/GurmitSingh/Papers/1317645/Are_we_missing_the_potential_of_action_research_for_transformative_change_in_medical_education

Schraw, G., & Dennison, R. S. (1994). Assessing metacognitive awareness. *Contemporary Educational Psychology, 19*(4), 460–475.

Shapiro, J., Rucker, L., & Beck, J. (2006). Training the clinical eye and mind: Using the arts to develop medical students' observational and pattern recognition skills. *Medical Education, 40*(3), 263–268.

Stringer, E. (2004). *Action research in education.* Upper Saddle River, NJ: Pearson Education.

Walter, J. M (2013). *Technologies of Nursing Practice (course).* Virginia Commonwealth University. Blackboard: http://blackboard.vcu.edu

Wikström, B. (2000). The development of observational competence through identification of nursing care patterns in 'The Sickbed,' a work of art by Lena Cronqvist. *Journal of Interprofessional Care, 14*(2), 181–188.

Wilson McKay, S., & Monteverde, S. (2003). Dialogic looking: Beyond the mediated experience. *Art Education: The Journal of the National Art Education Association, 56*(1), 40–45. Available from http://www.jstor.org/stable/3194031

World Health Organization. (2010). *Framework for action on interprofessional education & collaborative practice.* Geneva, Switzerland: Author. Available from http://whqlibdoc.who.int/hq/2010/WHO_HRH_HPN_10.3_eng.pdf

# The NLN Center for Innovation in Simulation and Technology

# 17

# Team-Based Learning in Online Nursing Education: An Innovation in Curriculum Development

**Kathleen M. Gambino,** EdD, RN
**Carol B. Della Ratta,** PhD, CCRN
**Brenda L. Janotha,** DNP-DCC, ANP-BC, APRN
**Virginia A. Coletti,** PhD, RN, NPP, CS, CARN
**Terri A. Cavaliere,** DNP, RN, NNP-BC

Today's nursing workplace is increasingly complex, posing multiple challenges and requiring higher levels of competencies for new nurse graduates. Innovative teaching strategies that develop clinical reasoning and collaborative skills must be an integral part of the nursing curricula to assist in the transition to this fast-paced, transdisciplinary environment. To that end, faculty are exploring teaching strategies that provide classroom opportunities for students to fully engage and assume shared accountability for learning (Clark, Nguyen, Bray, & Levine, 2008; Hickman & Wocial, 2013).

Team-based learning (TBL) is a multiphase pedagogical approach requiring active student participation and collaboration. This unique educational platform is designed to enhance learning through the interaction of high-performing teams (Michaelsen, Knight, & Fink, 2008). Evidence of improved student outcomes associated with TBL has been attributed to a shift from passive learning to a more active and constructive process (Grady, 2011). Moreover, active student participation is valued because of its far-reaching potential in providing lifelong learning skills (Li, An, & Li, 2010) and in developing the clinical reasoning skills needed to analyze and solve complex patient problems (Hickman & Wocial, 2013). TBL is composed of three stages (Michaelson et al.):

1. Pre-lesson activities that are completed by individual students

2. In-class learning assurance assessments with instructor feedback

3. Team discussion assignments that promote application of course content and assess team mastery of subject matter

Team discussion assignments should adhere to what is known as the "4S's" (Michaelsen et al., 2008):

1. *Significant* to the student
2. The *Same* for all teams
3. Require that a *Specific* choice be made
4. Reported *Simultaneously*

TBL strategies were introduced in the onsite classrooms of a northeastern public university school of nursing, but they were not used in the school's online learning program. The goal for implementing TBL in the school's online program was to enhance learning and foster the development of collaborative skills in a geographically diverse population of students. With this goal in mind, revisions were made to an existing asynchronous online undergraduate research course offered in an RN baccalaureate program or RN-to-BSN program.

## COURSE DESIGN AND REVISION

Previously, the online course consisted of lectures, assigned readings, and collaborative worksheets. An individually submitted research critique paper and an end-of-semester multiple choice final exam were additional requirements. Worksheets were completed by student-selected groups of approximately five individuals. Each student's contribution was identified by varying-colored font. However, as with many online programs, faculty had observed a lack of true collaborative effort among the group members, as revealed by responses on worksheets, student feedback, individual paper grades, and final exam scores. Implementation of a pedagogical approach that would promote self-directed learning, teamwork, and critical thinking was needed.

The revised course consisted of five TBL modules, each of which included an Individual Readiness Assurance Test (IRAT), a Group Readiness Assurance Test (GRAT), a Team Discussion Activity, and a peer evaluation. The five modules accounted for 55 percent of the total grade, and the remaining 45 percent was determined by an individually submitted research critique paper. The purpose of readiness assurance tests was to ensure individual student accountability. Students prepared for each module by completing the reading assignments and reviewing the PowerPoint® lectures provided. Each module included a 10-item multiple choice, closed-book IRAT that was to be completed in 10 minutes, within a predetermined 24-hour period. The next day, the teams were given the GRAT to complete in 1 week. The GRAT was composed of the same questions as the IRAT. The students were required to explain how they came to the answer they chose using their designated font color. The GRAT was graded on the team's final multiple choice selection, not on the discussion points. Throughout the semester, mini-critiques of research studies, assigned for the purpose of applying course principles and assessing mastery of content, served as team discussion activities. These activities adhered to three of the 4 S's:

1. *Significant* to the student (this skill is an essential first step in evidence-based nursing practice)
2. The *Same* for all teams (all teams received the same assignment)
3. Require that a *Specific* choice be made (questions posed required a specific choice, thus facilitating deeper analysis)

# IMPLEMENTATION OF THE COURSE

The course was implemented in spring 2014. Four online sections were created within the school's learning management system, with a total of 80 students enrolled. The courses were identical with regard to content, requirements, and deadline dates. Each of the faculty members from the Undergraduate Department who had revised the course taught one of the sections.

Students adapted to the TBL curriculum without requiring an excessive amount of guidance. This was attributed to the in-depth explanation of TBL principles presented in video and narrative format, as well as journal articles provided during the course introduction. Faculty responded to student concerns in a timely manner, taking into consideration that many students were adjusting to this unique pedagogical approach as they returned to academia for the first time in several years. Students gave positive feedback, and although the IRATs were difficult, as evidenced by individual grades ($M = 78.7$), teams consistently scored very well on the GRATS ($M = 98.1$). Furthermore, enhanced learning was evident in the final individually submitted research critique papers; students' grades were higher ($M = 90.8$) than expected and of better quality than written assignments from the previous online course ($M = 84.6$). Increased student accountability, inherent to TBL, resulted in improved engagement when completing individual and team assignments. Peer evaluations, an essential component of TBL (Michaelsen et al., 2008), provided the faculty with greater insight regarding individual online students. Attrition rates for the TBL online courses were similar to those of traditional onsite or online programs, with a total of four students dropping the course throughout the semester.

Although the online TBL course was successful, its introduction was not without problems. Some of the issues faced reflected those typical of many online courses, whereas others were unique to the online TBL curriculum. Assigning teams was one obstacle. Formulating heterogeneous teams of five to seven members who had no previous social contact (Michaelsen et al., 2008) was difficult because little was known about existing relationships among individuals enrolled in this course. Reviewing student demographic information was also a time-consuming process. Because the student population at this public university was diverse and it was unlikely this group of first-semester students had previous contact, three of the faculty decided to assign teams alphabetically. One instructor chose to formulate teams using student prerequisite grade point averages (GPAs), to equally distribute the intellectual capability. As recommended by Michaelsen et al., student teams remained permanent for the semester to optimize communication and function. Interestingly, student issues, performance on IRAT/GRAT, and final grades for each section indicated no differences in teams placed by GPA or by alphabetical assignment.

As often noted in other online courses, without the benefit of face-to-face interactions, communication and accountability issues arose. To address these issues, strictly enforced deadline dates were established for each required activity. Students who did not complete an IRAT by the deadline date received a failing grade for that assignment. As recommended by Parmelee and Michaelsen (2010), peer evaluation was used to facilitate team accountability by providing an opportunity for individuals to indicate how well other team members had contributed to their learning. Those who did not contribute to the GRAT or team discussion activities often received low peer evaluation scores from team members; this score was included in the final grade. As a result, students rarely missed a deadline as the semester progressed.

Using a computer-based system presented its own set of issues. Students occasionally would be "bumped off" the system while completing an IRAT, resulting in a delay from several hours to a full day, before it could be reset for completion. Originally, GRATs were to be released the day immediately following the IRAT submission date. Given that the IRAT and GRAT contained the same questions, it sometimes became necessary to postpone the release of the GRAT. To resolve this problem in the future, GRATs will be posted 2 days after the due date for the corresponding IRAT.

Adhering to the fourth "S," simultaneous team reporting was not possible in this asynchronous platform. As a result, the energetic exchanges noted in on-site TBL classes could not occur in the online course. In the future, using a discussion board and assigned posting time may allow for enhanced engagement among online teams.

Finally, despite detailed instructions and emails between faculty and students, the peer evaluation process was not consistently completed correctly. Some students were confused about the total number of points to allocate to team members, and others did not provide supporting statements with the number score as required by Michaelsen et al. (2008). Moreover, when student feedback was provided, it did not always coincide with the points allocated. As the course progressed and additional instructions were given, students began to submit appropriate peer evaluations. However, determination of the final peer evaluation grades was complicated by issues faced at the beginning of the semester. The wording of the peer evaluation instructions will be revised for future classes in an attempt to better explain the assignment and process.

## IMPLICATIONS FOR NURSING EDUCATION

Incorporating TBL into an online nursing research course enhanced students' learning through increased engagement and communication. Worksheets and team discussion activity responses provided evidence of self-directed learning, leading to improved discussions and collaboration among team members. Fostering these qualities in the distance nursing classroom was viewed positively by both the students and faculty. Most importantly, these skills may segue to improved critical thinking and higher-quality nursing care. A suggestion for future study is to examine learning outcomes of TBL pedagogy.

### References

Clark, M. C., Nguyen, H. T., Bray, C., & Levine, R. E. (2008). Team-based learning in an undergraduate nursing course. *Journal of Nursing Education, 47*(3), 111–117.

Grady, S. (2011). Team-based learning in pharmacotherapeutics. *American Journal of Pharmaceutical Education, 75*(7), 136.

Hickman, S. E., & Wocial, L. D. (2013). Team-based learning and ethics education in nursing. *Journal of Nursing Education, 52*(12), 696–700.

Li, L., An, L., & Li, W. (2010). Nursing students' self-directed learning. *Chinese General Nursing, 8*(5), 1205–1206.

Michaelsen, L., Knight, A. B., & Fink, L. D. (Eds.). (2008) *Team-based learning: A transformative use of small groups in college teaching.* Sterling, VA: Stylus Publishing.

Parmelee, D. X., & Michaelsen, L. K. (2010). Twelve tips for doing effective team-based learning (TBL). *Medical Teacher, 32*(2), 118–122.

# 18

# Incorporating Virtual Simulation into Undergraduate Education

**Karen A. Landry,** PhD, RN
**Mary Kathryn Sanders,** MSN, RN
**Renee T. Ridley,** PhD, RN
**Regina Bentley,** EdD, RN, CNE

Imagine a world for nursing students where they explore concepts discussed in class and practice the skills learned in lab to assess and treat patients. This world exists only for their learning needs, providing the promise that no harm will be done. Now imagine that students in this world actually converse with vulnerable patients, such as the mentally ill and even children, learning how best to communicate with and manage nursing care of these special populations. This world for students actually exists in the form of virtual simulation and can ease their transition from classroom to clinical. Multiuser virtual environments (MUVEs), such as Second Life® (SL), allow students to submerge themselves into areas of clinical experiential learning. This chapter will describe the process of incorporating SL into mental health and pediatric courses in an undergraduate BSN program.

SL is a computer-based virtual world owned by Linden Lab. It first became available to the public in 2003 on the Internet. Participants or users create avatars to move around the environment and interact with other users. The participants can speak and move objects. Users can purchase virtual private islands, land, homes, and items within SL from Linden Lab or another user. For example, purchasing a grid allows the individual to construct a virtual environment. Corporations, government, schools, and universities have used this environment to develop innovative properties used in showcasing products, information about certain diseases, and educational environments. These entities can buy a virtual island and create a virtual environment to meet their needs. This might include displaying the latest products or, in the case of education, simulating real-life situations in a virtual world.

The use of SL in both on-site and online nursing education has been shown to improve creative learning and decision-making skills, giving students the perception that they are more capable in the clinical setting (McCallum, Ness, & Price, 2011; Stewart et al., 2010). Students also claim that SL provides a safe, nonthreatening and positive environment, where they can role-play and practice skills, such as effective interview techniques (Aebersold,

Tschannen, Stephens, Anderson, & Lei, 2011; McCallum et al.; Stewart et al.; Sweigart, Hodson-Carlton, Campbell, & Lutz, 2010). SL, as a technology tool and experiential learning resource for students who learn best through kinesthetic modalities, has proven to be a positive simulation experience (Schmidt & Stewart, 2010). In general, students appreciate the real-time aspect and immediate feedback that SL allows (Schmidt & Stewart). To better assure these outcomes, faculty and students have identified the need for orientation to technology, strong technological support, clear expectations and explanations, specific avatar naming guidelines, professional dress requirements, and strategic curricular placement of SL simulations prior to actual face-to-face interactions in the real world (Schmidt & Stewart; Sweigart et al.).

Successful incorporation of SL into nursing education has been reported for community health, mental health, and pediatric courses, including simulations regarding long-term care, patient falls, public health issues, social justice, and disaster preparedness (Skiba, 2009; Stewart et al., 2010). Conversely, there is a learning curve for faculty who may feel intimidated by the technology aspect of SL. As well, there are barriers to easy access of SL environments that are already developed. For example, one study identified only 7 unique simulations for nursing education out of 29 communities that currently exist (Trangenstein, Weiner, Gordon, & McNew, 2010). This could indicate that in some universities, SL nursing education is closed to the public for copyright protection.

## NEED TO IMPLEMENT SECOND LIFE

Clinical sites for mental health and pediatrics are seasonal in central Texas, proving to be inadequate during times when nursing programs are growing and qualified faculty scarce. In an attempt to "think outside the box" for clinical experiences in nursing education, faculty of the college of nursing (CON) in a large university focused on a project to incorporate synchronous virtual simulations in mental health and pediatric undergraduate BSN courses. SL was chosen because it provides a virtual simulation experience using technology with which many students are familiar. This educational tool is facilitated by faculty but driven by students. SL allows faculty members to provide a variety of virtual clinical simulations while maintaining a consistent, safe experience for each student. It provides an alternate solution to ease clinical placement of students in areas that have limited available sites. Implementation of these simulations not only would fill the need for specialized patient encounters but also would incorporate the use of the electronic health record (EHR), providing a creative way for students to experience nursing informatics across the curriculum. Navigating through a live EHR would prepare students for current healthcare expectations and guidelines.

## COLLABORATION EFFORTS

In August and September 2010, the project directors, with support and assistance from the CON administration, invited key nursing leaders in surrounding communities to become part of the Second Life Advisory Committee (SLAC). This committee advised the project directors and was required as part of a grant received by the CON for project implementation. Most of these leaders accepted the invitation either to serve on the committee or designated individuals from their organizations who had a special interest in nursing education, especially innovative teaching methods. Members of the SLAC included nursing educators, hospital administration leaders, and directors of nursing programs. The SLAC, comprised of 12 members, met a total of three times. The committee discussed updates on the grant, made suggestions on improving the design of the virtual simulation environment, and gave recommendations for content experts to help in the development of scenarios.

## STRATEGY

Planning began almost immediately for the Virtual Simulation in Nursing Clinical Instruction project after notification of a grant award in 2010. Approval for data collection from students was obtained from the IRB. Meetings were initiated with the university's vice president for Program Development and Community Outreach, the dean and associate dean for the CON, local community college nursing administration, university and community college nursing faculty, and the SL designers to develop strategies for creating virtual hospital clinical scenarios and partnerships. The university purchased two islands specifically designated for the development of the virtual pediatric and mental health hospitals.

## PROJECT OBJECTIVES

The expected outcomes/objectives of incorporating SL into undergraduate education were to:

1. Develop a virtual hospital containing detailed pediatric and mental health units.
2. Create eight high-quality case scenarios (four pediatric and four mental health).
3. Increase nursing students' knowledge about pediatric and mental health concepts and skills.
4. Enroll a minimum of 25 percent more nursing students in the CON as a result of implementing simulated clinical experiences in SL for pediatric and mental health courses.
5. Provide additional clinical experiences for the local community college, which had recently increased its numbers.

For the purpose of this chapter, only objectives 1 and 2 will be addressed. Objectives 3, 4, and 5 will be discussed in a follow-up.

## CREATING SECOND LIFE RESOURCES

Resources were extremely important for the foundation of this project. Distinctive SL designers were chosen for the project, those specializing in a particular design area. One designer created the physical structures on each island, and the second designer developed the programing. Purchase of the islands was necessary prior to the start of

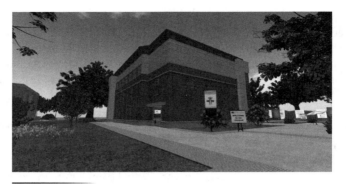

**FIGURE 18.1** TAMHSC College of Nursing in Second Life. Used with permission of Texas A&M Health Science Center, College of Nursing.

construction. Special SL orientation resources were needed for faculty, students, and standardized patients (SPs). The project directors created explicit manuals to address the needs of the different areas. The manuals explain how to create an avatar, participate in a scavenger hunt, tour the SL hospital, and participate in a mock scenario.

## HOSPITAL DESIGN

Design and creation of the virtual hospitals were completed over a period of 1 year. The hospitals are located on two SL islands and are restricted to the public, allowing protection of the learning environment. Outer portions of the buildings resemble brick and mortar, designed as replications of the university campus. Plants, trees, and fountains are used to decorate the lobby areas (Figure 18.1).

The pediatric hospital has an emergency center and unit. This allows for scenarios to be created over a greater variety of acuity. The emergency center and pediatric unit both contain five pediatric treatment rooms. The rooms in the pediatric unit are decorated with childlike themes and bright colors. Every room in both the emergency center and unit includes a bed or crib (depending on the scenario), cardiac monitor, overhead lighting, nightstands and side tables, bathrooms, furniture (table and multiple chairs), a writing desk with chair, closet, sharps container, sink with running water, soap, towels, and trash cans. Outside of each patient's room is a hand sanitizer dispenser. Within the hallways are wheelchairs and stretchers, isolation carts, and crash carts. The patients' rooms are designed so that conversations are only heard in each of the rooms (Figure 18.2). A curtain is used to close the front of the patient's room to ensure privacy.

There are at least two interprofessional healthcare (IPH) stations (similar to nursing stations) located on each unit. They too are designated as "private areas," allowing for confidentiality within the virtual clinical environment. The IPH stations contain computers so that the healthcare team can chart within the EHR as needed. A "live" EHR was selected for this project. The EHR requires students to document and gives faculty the opportunity to evaluate each student's work, providing appropriate feedback. EHR kiosks are located next to medication dispensing machines outside each patient's room in the pediatric areas and within the IPH stations on the mental health unit.

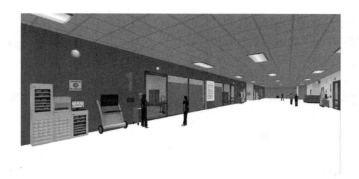

**FIGURE 18.2** TAMHSC Pediatric Hospital Patient Unit in Second Life. Used with permission of Texas A&M Health Science Center, College of Nursing.

Within the mental health virtual clinical area, there are sleeping areas and interviewing areas. The interviewing areas are equipped with large nonbreakable windows and heavy tables/chairs. Beside every patient's room or interview room is a faculty observation room. This room allows faculty to observe student interactions with the patient and/or a parent without interrupting the conversation. Rooms are not soundproof, so silence is cautioned. Students are aware that faculty may observe in this manner. Each room also contains a tracking screen where each student's interventions can be tracked chronologically. At the end of the scenario, this information is automatically sent to the faculty member, allowing faculty to provide critical feedback to students on their clinical performance for that day.

Within each hospital are sitting areas, medication-dispensing devices, kiosks that provide viewing of the EHR, IPH stations, and conference areas. Telephones are located on the wall outside of each patient's room to allow students to call for needed services within the hospital.

## SCENARIOS

Four pediatric and four mental health clinical scenarios, learning modules, and pre- and post-tests were developed in collaboration with content experts. Pediatric content consists of asthma, RSV bronchiolitis, bacterial meningitis, and Kawasaki's disease. Also developed for each scenario was a learning module, allowing students to review a particular disease process prior to the clinical day. Pre- and post-tests were developed to measure knowledge before and after the learning experience. In addition, a grading rubric to evaluate clinical performances was created for each scenario.

Each scenario was developed to include the following:

- Brief overview
- Essential core concepts
- Student learning objective
- Level (beginning, intermediate, or complex)

- SL simulation site
- Recommended student group size
- Patient description
- Student responsibilities prior to simulation
- Scenario staging (environment, equipment, supplies, and avatar descriptions)
- Actors in scenario
- Pre-scenario briefing (students)
- Scenario progression script
- Post-scenario activities

Each scenario is embedded with the Quality and Safety Education for Nurses (QSEN) safety guidelines, National Council of State Boards of Nursing (NCLEX) blueprint, and Texas Board of Nursing (TBON) Differentiated Essential Competencies (DECs) of Graduates of Texas Nursing Programs for both ADN and BSN programs.

## AVATARS

Students and faculty created their own avatars for use in this project. Students had specific rules to follow concerning the design of their avatars. For example, student avatars must be human, wear short hair or ponytail, and be in school uniform. A uniform store located in the university administration building allows students to choose the school's uniform. The project designers and SL designers created specific patient and/or parent avatars for use in each scenario. For example, an avatar that represents a patient's role has been created for each scenario (Figure 18.3). Team members secure all usernames and passwords to protect the restricted area. Each avatar is dressed the same and can be morphed into either male or female. Depending on the scenario, the parent avatar may also be used. There are additional players in the script, such as a nurse, healthcare provider, or healthcare worker. Because there are five patient rooms in each clinical rotation, five patient avatars are used. A positive feature about virtual clinical simulation is the use

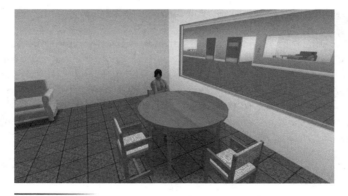

**FIGURE 18.3** TAMHSC Mental Health Hospital Patient Unit in Second Life. Used with permission of Texas A&M Health Science Center, College of Nursing.

of culturally diverse avatars. This feature allows students to experience and learn about different cultures.

## STANDARDIZED PATIENTS

SPs are used in each scenario. These individuals are trained to play a role within the scenario as a patient or parent. Something that must be considered with using SPs in virtual simulation is their ability to use a computer. Although the amount of computer knowledge needed is minimal, it is necessary. SPs have a 2-hour orientation in the use of SL that includes using the speak function. Each SP follows a script for each scenario.

## VIRTUAL CLINICAL EXPERIENCE: PUTTING IT ALL TOGETHER

The preparation for each semester starts months ahead of implementing this simulation. Approximately a week prior to the virtual simulation clinical experience, students have the opportunity to view the learning module for that particular scenario. Prior to the clinical day, project directors prepare schedules; reserve rooms; and secure computers, students, and faculty. Learning modules were developed by faculty members, and each incorporate creative pictures and designs that ease reading and facilitate learning.

The content within each module is:

- Essential core concepts related to the learning module
- Expected student outcomes
- Supporting textbook references
- Discussion about specific diseases
- Assessment
- Nursing interventions
- Drug therapies
- References

On clinical day, the faculty member meets students in SL for a pre-scenario briefing. Typically, faculty and students gather in the conference room of the university CON building. At any time, the faculty member may take students to the third floor practice area. This area is an exact duplicate of a pediatric hospital room or mental health inter-view room. Students are able to travel the virtual floors via elevator. Upon completion of this briefing, students move to a "learning resource center." Here, a learning module for the specific scenario is posted for their review. After students complete these activities, they walk to the "testing center."

This area is private and soundproof to provide a secure area for proctoring the test. Students walk to a stool and sit down within the testing center. Once seated, a prompt screen allows the student to choose which test to take (pre/post). Each test has 10 multi-ple choice questions. There is parallel construction of pre- and post-tests. In other words, the questions are not the same for each test; however, the concepts are. For example, disease-specific pathophysiology, medication knowledge, nursing interventions, and so forth, would be incorporated into each test. After completion of the test, the results are sent to the designated faculty member. Each student completes a pre-test prior to the virtual clinical simulation experience. After all students have completed the test, they progress to the virtual clinical simulation area in the mental health or pediatric hospital.

Within the pediatric experience, students walk onto the unit and are assigned a pediatric patient by the faculty member. Students are allowed to go to a kiosk on the unit (there are several) to access the EHR. After reviewing the EHR, students begin interacting with the patient and/or parent. Students are able to complete detailed assessments with actual audio sounds and have active interaction with the patient and/or parent. There are cardiac monitors in every room with live data for students to interpret. Along with the faculty member, students administer medications. Many nursing interventions take place, such as patient assessments, patient/parent teaching, medication administration, and measuring vital signs. Students must critically think and use decision-making processes based on their knowledge of the specific disease process used in the specific scenario.

Students and faculty have the opportunity to interact with other healthcare professionals within the scenarios. This interaction is a great opportunity to integrate interprofessional education into the virtual clinical environment. For example, pharmacy students are able to help with inputting data and virtual medications within the medication administration devices, and medical students can help with medical procedures and writing orders.

Upon completing the virtual clinical scenario, which includes giving report to the primary nurse, faculty and students meet in the virtual conference room for debriefing of the clinical day's events. Following debriefing, students end their day with a post-test.

Within the mental health virtual clinical experience, students have similar experiences with the pre-scenario briefing, learning resource center, pre- and post-test, EHR, IPH stations, and conference space. However, the student learning outcomes primarily focus on therapeutic communication and client and psychosocial assessments. Therefore, students enter the hospital through a secured door into an area where patients are sitting in rooms waiting for an interview.

## LESSONS LEARNED

One mental health and four pediatric scenarios were used during the fall 2011 and spring 2012 semesters. Seven faculty members and 144 students participated in the project. Lessons learned were valuable to advance knowledge of teaching modalities within the clinical environment. During virtual clinical experiences in SL, technology support for students and faculty members (i.e., troubleshooting sound) was critical to the project's success. Organization of faculty and student orientation, as well as clinical schedules, was also important. Faculty/student orientation included creating avatars, introducing students to the virtual hospitals, and maneuvering documentation in the EHR. Time spent in orientation saved valuable clinical simulation time and resulted in scenarios running smoothly.

Early on, a great detail of effort was put into the creation of each simulation experience. Scenarios were scripted with details about acute and chronic illnesses. A full year was needed to develop virtual hospitals and the eight simulation scenarios.

Virtual clinical simulations were strategically placed within the clinical rotations based on student feedback. For mental health, the virtual clinical simulation experience was placed at the beginning of the semester. This allowed students to enhance therapeutic communication skills prior to entering into an actual hospital environment. Feedback from students concerning the pediatric virtual clinical simulation, however, showed that they preferred the experience toward the end of clinical rotations.

Making sure that students and SPs had the physical space needed to conduct virtual clinical simulations was essential. It became necessary to ensure privacy for students and SPs when they were conducting synchronous communication within the virtual hospital experience. Either individual rooms or a large room separated by individual curtains provided for such privacy.

## CONCLUSION

Virtual clinical experiences give unlimited opportunities in nursing education. The first objective for this project was developing a virtual hospital containing detailed pediatric and mental health units. A summary was provided on ways to create a virtual hospital offering valued clinical experiences for institutions interested in exploring new ways to conduct virtual clinical experiences. For future projects, interprofessional education will be addressed. This type of venue provides an excellent opportunity and platform for such a design. The second objective for this project was creating eight high-quality case scenarios (four pediatric and four mental health) for SL use. This objective was met.

The next phase of this project will be extending the virtual clinical experience to maternal-child, community, and medical-surgical areas. Moreover, further use of the EHR will be supported. Virtual clinical experiences incorporating interprofessional collaboration will be pursued. This platform allows for students to join the scenario from different campuses. Faculty can also join in from desktop computers within their offices.

Long-term viability of the project will depend on primary support. Linden Lab recently made changes to its business model. This change has affected academia by increasing the cost needed to set up virtual learning environments in SL. In the past, schools and universities received a discount. Although this decision has been disappointing and perhaps a setback for some programs, faculty should seek alternative ways to secure funding for future SL projects.

Another frequently asked question concerns transferability or copyrights. Transferability is possible within SL. However, at this time, the university has no intention of transferring any virtual environment. In fact, plans for expansion are in progress. Purchase of the nursing environment concept is possible with respect to acquiring permission, copyright adherence, and SL rights. However, to support such an endeavor, strong technical support, as well as nurse educator consultation for orientation and implementation, should be seriously considered.

The future of virtual clinical experiences is promising and can add to the body of knowledge for nursing education. Challenges should be examined and costs assessed. Virtual clinical simulation provides a unique way of providing clinical education and allows the opportunity to capture creative experiential learning that can cultivate nurses of tomorrow.

## References

Aebersold, M., Tschannen, D., Stephens, M., Anderson, P., & Lei, X. (2011). Second Life®: A new strategy in educating nursing students. *Clinical Simulation in Nursing, 8*(9), e469–e475.

McCallum, J., Ness, V., & Price, T. (2011). Exploring nursing students' decision-making skills whilst in a Second Life® clinical simulation laboratory. *Nurse Education Today, 31*(7), 699–704.

Schmidt, B., & Stewart, S. (2010). Implementing the virtual world of Second Life® into community nursing theory and clinical courses. *Nurse Educator, 35*(2), 74–78.

Skiba, D. (2009). Nursing education 2.0: A second look at Second Life®. *Nursing Education Perspectives, 30*(2), 129–131.

Stewart, S., Hansen, T., Pope, D., Schmidt, B., Thyes, J., Jambunathan, J., et al. (2010). Developing a Second Life® campus for online accelerated BSN students. *CIN: Computers, Informatics, Nursing, 28*(5), 253–258.

Sweigart, L., Hodson-Carlton, K., Campbell, B., & Lutz, D. (2010). Second Life® environment: A venue for interview skill development. *CIN: Computers, Informatics, Nursing, 28*(5), 258–263.

Trangenstein, P., Weiner, E., Gordon, J., & McNew, R. (2010). An analysis of nursing education's immersion into Second Life®, a multi-user virtual environment (MUVE). *Studies in Health Technology & Informatics, 160*(Pt. 1), 644–647.

# 19

# Innovative Web 2.0 Teaching Tool: GoAnimate

**Kezia D. Lilly,** DNP, MBA HC, RN
**Dana Hunt,** DNP, MPH, RN

New Web 2.0 technology tools are redefining higher education. A university faculty member introduced an innovative Web 2.0 technology called *GoAnimate* during a DNP intensive. This chapter introduces GoAnimate and ways that GoAnimate can be used in nursing education, and provides a pilot survey that explored student perceptions of using this as a teaching tool.

Technology continues to drive change in online nursing education. Technological innovation has a major influence on teaching methods and is a core differentiator in attracting students (Robina & Anderson, 2010).

As new technologies redefine literacy in higher education, nurse educators need to look for teaching strategies to accommodate 21st-century, tech-savvy learners (Smith & Dobson, 2011). GoAnimate was used at Case Western Reserve University (CWRU) to deliver course objectives in a DNP program.

## WEB 2.0

According to Harris, Barden, Walker, and Reznek (2009), a successful curriculum will have integrated technology that places students at the center of learning. Student learning has been shown to increase with the use of Web 2.0 tools (Lemley & Burnham, 2009; Smith & Dobson, 2011), collaborative tools that include blogs, podcasts, wikis, and photosharing (Lemley & Burnham). Web 2.0 tools are an easy and inexpensive way to engage students in the learning experience (Imperatore, 2009).

A study by Lemley and Burnham (2009) found that only 53 percent of nursing schools used Web 2.0 tools, and these were used primarily in graduate and leadership curricula. To increase knowledge and enhance technology in health care, it is important that nursing institutions recognize, revise, and advance nursing curricula to include the use of Web 2.0 tools (Glasgow, Dunphy, & Mainous, 2010).

## GoAnimate

GoAnimate (http://goanimate.com/about) is an innovative Web 2.0 tool that allows faculty and students to simulate and animate nursing scenes through creatively staged information. Scenes in GoAnimate are similar to slides in PowerPoint. The software allows the user to create animated videos quickly and easily, selecting or building a variety of settings, characters, props, animations, audio, and narration.

The free version of GoAnimate allows up to five minutes of animated videos, whereas the professional version allows unlimited videos for $18 per quarter hour. In nursing education, GoAnimate can be used to create role-playing scenarios, present controversial topics and case studies, and create simulations for pre-licensure or graduate nursing programs.

Four DNP students taking part in an intensive course at CWRU used GoAnimate software to present a curriculum development proposal for a nursing program. The assignment required a group presentation on the development of the curriculum with a philosophy, organizational framework, program outcomes, and major threads and concepts. GoAnimate characters were used to represent each of the students with a personalized audio for each student, visuals that included a PowerPoint presentation as a background prop, and supplemental handouts. Table 19.1 provides the link to this GoAnimate presentation and others using various technologies.

A pilot survey was submitted to the participating class to evaluate how students responded to the GoAnimate presentation. The respondents (half of those eligible to participate) included three students in a master's program, three in the doctoral program, and one DNP professor.

All respondents reported that they had not previously been exposed to GoAnimate. Of the respondents, nine reported that they would consider using this teaching method now that they had been exposed to the software. All respondents reported that they enjoyed the content delivery using this method. Comments received about the teaching method included, "fun way to get information across," "brought humor into the classroom," and "it was a great teaching tool; I look forward to using it." Respondents planned to use GoAnimate to show students both poor and exemplar situations, create role-playing situations, and encourage students to use the program for presentations.

Following the DNP course, fellow classmates, peers, and colleagues have used GoAnimate to deliver staff training, course assignments, instructional strategies, regional and state conferences, and information videos. Examples are included in Table 19.1.

## CONCLUSION

As a profession, nursing is still learning how to respond to the challenge of educating students to use new technologies. As found during our classroom experience in a DNP program, students and educators, regardless of age, enjoy new and innovative teaching strategies that are effective in enhancing learning. With technology being a driving force in higher education, we must seek out and share our teaching strategies, and administrators in schools of nursing will need to provide educational resources to support educators in learning these new teaching tools.

## TABLE 19.1

## Links to GoAnimate and Other Technology Presentations

| Name of Presentation | URL | Creator | Description/Purpose |
|---|---|---|---|
| NUND 509 RUMBA University RN-BSN Curriculum | http://goanimate.com/videos/0FSxt2uWsRjo?utm_source=linkshare | Kezia Lilly and contributors: Cozi Bagley, Rebecca Patton, Vanessa Lelli | During a DNP intensive for a curriculum course, a group assignment required students to present a curriculum plan. |
| Missouri Society of Radiologic Technologists State Conference 2013 | http://goanimate.com/videos/07482oiv-BKY?utm_source=linkshare&utm_medium=linkshare&utm_campaign=usercontent | Kezia Lilly, Stacy Soden | GoAnimate was introduced as a teaching strategy. |
| Changing Your Servix Through EBP | http://goanimate.com/videos/0foo4cLf9iJM?utm_source=linkshare | Cozi Bagley | Staff development for evidence-based practice, one-on-one patient to nurse care in labor and delivery. |
| SBU Faculty Dev Audacity Tutorial | http://goanimate.com/videos/0zJLaH1qeBvA?utm_source=linkshare | Kezia Lilly and contributors: Dana Hunt, Terri Schmitt, Stacy Soden | Faculty development to introduce Audacity. |
| Twitter Assignment | http://goanimate.com/videos/01D7cMHNW88Q?utm_source=linkshare | Kezia Lilly | Introduction of a BSN informatics course assignment, Twitter. |
| NUND 530 Research Problem | http://goanimate.com/videos/0ZDMXP5QcVEg?utm_source=linkshare | Kezia Lilly | During a DNP CWRU intensive, a research assignment required students to present their research problem to the class. |

## References

Glasgow, M. E. S., Dunphy, L. M., & Mainous, R. O. (2010). Innovative nursing educational curriculum for the 21st century nurse. *Nursing Education Perspectives, 31*(6), 355–357.

Harris, S. S., Barden, B., Walker, H. K., & Reznek, M. A. (2009). Assessment of student learning behaviors to guide the integration of technology in curriculum reform. *Informatics Services & Use, 29*(1), 45–52.

Imperatore, C. (2009). What you need to know about Web 2.0. *Techniques: Connecting Education and Careers, 84*(1), 20–23.

Lemley, T., & Burnham, J. (2009). Web 2.0 tools in medical and nursing school curricula. *Journal of the Medical Library Association, 97*(1), 50–52.

Robina, K., & Anderson, M. (2010). Online teaching efficacy of nurse faculty. *Journal of Professional Nursing, 26*(3), 168–175.

Smith, J., & Dobson, E. (2011). Beyond the book: Using Web 2.0 tools to develop 21st century literacies. *Computers in the Schools, 28*(4), 316–327.

# 20

# An Innovative Approach Using Clinical Simulation to Teach Quality and Safety Principles to Undergraduate Nursing Students

**Mary Ann Cantrell,** PhD, RN, CNE
**Bette Mariani,** PhD, RN
**Colleen H. Meakim,** MSN, RN, CHSE

Clinical simulation is an evidence-based teaching strategy that is used to teach safety-conscious practice behaviors among pre-licensure nursing professionals (Lasater, 2007; Mariani, Cantrell, Meakim, Prieto, & Dreifuerst, 2013; Shinnick, Woo, Horwich, & Steadman, 2011). Simulation is an emerging evidence-based teaching-learning strategy for undergraduate nursing students that provides opportunities for learners to make decisions in a safe environment, witness the consequences and evaluate the effectiveness of their actions, and demonstrate clinical judgment (Benner, Sutphen, Leonard, & Day, 2010; Sears, Goldsworthy, & Goodman, 2010). Recent trends in health care, the drive for safety and quality initiatives in healthcare systems, and the need to augment clinical and classroom experiences for students have driven the interest in, and support for, this growing pedagogy (Cronenwett et al., 2007; Henneman & Cunningham, 2009; Institute of Medicine, 2010).

The overall aim of this project was to enhance students' knowledge of safety principles using a three-fold simulated learning experience. The simulated learning experience involved viewing two prerecorded scenarios. One scenario was a suboptimal scenario in which safety practices were violated or ignored, and the other scenario was an optimal scenario in which safety practice behaviors were consistently demonstrated. The second aspect of the scenario was an assessment of the simulated scene in which students performed an environmental safety check. The final component of the learning experience was a formal debriefing session. The following learning objectives for the scenario were included:

1. Identify communication practices that minimize risks associated with handoffs and transitions of care.

2. Implement the nursing process to minimize patient safety risk.

3. Reflect upon how the nurse in a leadership role can promote a blame-free environment.

4. Describe how to delegate care interventions appropriately within the scope of practice for healthcare team members.

This project addressed three important aspects of simulation for undergraduate students:

1. Critical reasoning/judgment skills

2. Fidelity of the simulated learning experience to an actual patient experience

3. Incorporation of a model demonstration of the scenario.

The conceptual basis for this project was a teaching-learning strategy—What's Wrong With This Patient (WWWTP)—developed by Paparella, Mariani, Layton, and Carpenter (2004). This strategy required the learner to evaluate a simulated learning environment and identify what safety practices were not followed, then identify strategies to correct these errors. The WWWTP teaching strategy was extended in this project to have the learner evaluate the effectiveness of teamwork and collaboration, scope of practice, and appropriate role delegation among the healthcare team members.

An important aspect of this project was fidelity. Fidelity is defined as the degree to which the simulated learning experience depicts the real-life patient care situation it represents. The scenario for this simulated learning experience was based upon the actual experiences of a chronically ill young adult. An in-depth interview with a young adult with a chronic illness was conducted, and the information gleaned from this interview was used to construct the scenario. In addition, this young adult provided input and critique of the scenario, offering enhanced fidelity related to his own clinical care experiences. To further ensure fidelity of the simulated clinical experience, the role of the patient in the simulation was played by this young man.

An evidence-based strategy used in this teaching-learning experience was the incorporation of a model demonstration into the debriefing session that occurred at the conclusion of the experience. Cantrell (2008) conducted a focus group among eight students to understand the importance of debriefing following a simulated learning experience. Participants in Cantrell's study suggested that a scenario that accurately demonstrated nursing actions (a model demonstration) would significantly enhance their learning about the most effective behaviors a nurse would demonstrate in the scenario. For this project, a model demonstration of the patient care situation was video-taped and shared with students at the conclusion of the learning experience.

## DESCRIPTION OF THE TEACHING-LEARNING STRATEGY

The scenario for this clinical simulated experience involved a young adult male admitted to the hospital for an exacerbation of Crohn's disease. The scenario was developed using suggested teaching-learning strategies from the Quality and Safety in Nursing Education (QSEN) initiative. The scene depicts the patient lying in bed in pain; he has a central venous intravenous (IV) line with fluids infusing, and he is receiving an IV opioid via a patient-controlled analgesia (PCA) pump. Accompanying materials developed for the learning experience included:

1. Learning objectives
2. Preparation guidelines for students
3. Detailed account of the patient's physical and psychosocial history, as well as a complete account of his condition that required the hospital admission
4. Comprehensive list of materials and equipment needed for the scenario
5. I-SBAR report
6. List of behaviors to be demonstrated for the suboptimal and optimal scenario
7. List of care provider orders
8. Simulated environmental scenario observation checklist
9. Line-by-line script for both the suboptimal and optimal scenarios.

Table 20.1 depicts an excerpt from the same scene portrayed in the suboptimal and optimal scenarios.

This simulated learning activity was part of a study to assess students' learning and was embedded within the theory component of a leadership and management course for senior-level undergraduate nursing students. The project included 175 senior-level nursing students clustered into groups of 8 to 10 students per group. The learning experience was 75 minutes in duration. Institutional review board approval to conduct the study was received, and written consent was obtained from study participants. The following text outlines the learning experience in which students engaged in the following learning activities:

1. Completed a study guide that addressed the principles of communication, delegation, power, and conflict related to safe nursing practice that included a selected reading and a narrated PowerPoint® lecture on quality and safety issues in professional nursing practice
2. Evaluated a simulated setup of the patient environment that was a replication of the recorded scenario for safety features and potential high-risk elements, using a structured checklist
3. Viewed the prerecorded suboptimal scenario
4. Participated in a structured debriefing session, which focused on the at-risk safety practice behaviors and corrective actions and the leadership role of the nurse in the suboptimal scenario
5. Viewed the model demonstration of the scenario that demonstrated optimal practice behaviors (optimal scenario) at the conclusion of the debriefing session

## STUDENTS' PERCEPTIONS OF THE TEACHING-LEARNING EXPERIENCE

Approximately 2 weeks following this teaching-learning experience, students were invited to share feedback about their experiences by responding to four questions via

## TABLE 20.1

## Excerpt From a Scene Portrayed in the Suboptimal and Optimal Scenario

| Suboptimal Video Scene | Optimal Video Scene |
|---|---|
| 1. The patient rings his call bell, stating he is in pain. | 1. The patient rings his call bell, stating he is in pain. |
| 2. RN enters the room without washing hands. | 2. RN enters the room and immediately washes hands. |
| 3. RN briefly asks the patient why he rang the call bell and notices unlabeled lab specimens at the bedside and that the patient's central line dressing is peeling off. RN places a piece of tape over the existing dressing. RN leaves the lab specimens where she found them. | 3. RN addresses the patient and reminds him of her name and role. |
| | 4. RN completes a focused pain assessment that includes detailed questions about pain relief measures that have decreased the patient's pain previously. |
| 4. LPN is in the patient's room and is in the process of giving medications. LPN questions RN if she (LPN) should be giving the IV methylprednisolone. | 5. RN notes the patient's central line dressing is peeling off and takes appropriate action to have a fresh dressing applied by calling the IV team. |
| 5. RN tells LPN to go ahead and give the medication since she (RN) is in the room. | 6. RN notices unlabeled lab specimens at the bedside and removes the specimens from the patient's bedside. |
| 6. LPN notices the patient's ID band is missing. When questioned, the patient states he took it off last night because it was "itchy." RN states she will get someone to replace the ID band soon and instructs LPN to continue to administer the medication. | 7. LPN is in the patient's room and is in the process of giving medications. LPN questions RN if she (LPN) should be giving the IV medication. RN states that is her (RN's) responsibility and that she will administer the medication after checking the dose. |
| 7. RN notices the patient's bed is raised off the floor from the lowest position. The patient states he likes it that way. RN says that is fine if he wants to keep it raised for his convenience. | 8. LPN notices the patient's ID band is missing. When questioned, the patient states he took it off last night because it was "itchy." RN instructs LPN to leave the room and to return with an ID band that will be placed on the patient's wrist. |
| 8. RN reviews the PCA pump and notes the pump was turned off for a short period during the night. RN says something about it being off to LPN and the patient but does no further follow-up actions. | 9. RN notices the patient's bed is raised off the floor from the lowest position. The patient states he likes it that way. RN shares with the patient that keeping the bed in the lowest position is best safety practice and lowers the bed. |
| 9. The patient complains of pain again. RN is hesitant to administer an additional dose of a narcotic (rescue dose) and questions if the pain is in his abdomen or if the pain is related to fatigue and/or emotional stress. | 10. RN reviews the PCA pump and notes the pump was turned off for a short period during the night; she then completes an event report and she places a request for new machine. |
| 10. RN then leaves the room without any additional follow-up assessments. | 11. RN further evaluates the pain and recognizes that PCA was off overnight and administers an additional dose of a narcotic (rescue dose). She completes an event report. |

an email response. The open-ended questions included: What aspects of this learning experience were most helpful? What would make the learning experience better? How did the videos, environmental survey, and/or debriefing contribute to learning? What leadership roles of the nurse were you able to identify related to quality and safety? Students positively perceived this learning experience to be a "hands-on" experience and a new way to learn. Students identified the most helpful aspects of this experience in their learning were:

1. Watching the optimal and suboptimal videos
2. Participating in the debriefing in which they heard other students' perceptions of the scenarios
3. Assessing the scene and completing the environmental survey, which provided them with an engaging, hands-on approach to learning

Students identified that the group discussion in the debriefing session was very helpful in improving their knowledge by using a team approach to identify errors in the suboptimal video and the simulated patient care scene. They believed that they learned by hearing others identify errors in the videos and in the simulated environment that they did not identify. Overall, students reported that the use of the three-fold approach of watching suboptimal and optimal video, participating in the structured debriefing, and observing the scene to assess the environment for safety issues complemented the learning and was an effective approach to learning. When asked what would make the learning experience better, students suggested that the scenarios include more types of errors and to have additional opportunities to view the optimal and suboptimal videos rather than just once. Finally, when asked if they were able to identify leadership roles of the nurse related to quality and safety, students believed that they were better prepared to identify situations that could jeopardize quality and safety, as well as perform environmental safety checks. They also understood that the nurse is a key person in ensuring quality and safe patient care. Students also shared that from this experience they better understood the nurse's role in delegation, the importance of acknowledging mistakes and reporting errors, teamwork and collaboration, sharing with the patient why certain practices are required to ensure patient safety, and maintaining a blame-free environment.

## LESSONS LEARNED

When asked what would make the learning experience more effective, students suggested that the scenarios should have included more types of errors and that more than one opportunity to view the optimal and suboptimal videos should have been provided. Posting the videos on an e-learning platform for longer student access should be considered. Additional safety errors and perhaps additional scenarios with a variety of patient care situations would enhance students' learning. The coordination of 175 students through all steps of the learning experience was time consuming and confusing for students. Students suggested that a more organized approach to implementing the experience would be to post signs outside the rooms with students' names and to designate the specific part of the learning experience that will occur, and at what time and for how long students should be participating in this step of the learning experience.

# CONCLUSION

This project used the interactive, student-centered learning strategies of WWWTP and structured debriefing within a simulated learning experience to enhance students' understanding and awareness of safety practice behaviors within the context of the nurse leadership role. The conceptualization of the project was built upon evidence from the findings of past studies in the areas of debriefing and simulation. The use of a model demonstration was positively received by the students who participated in this project.

## *References*

Benner, P., Sutphen, M., Leonard, V., & Day, L. (2010). *Educating nurses: A call for radical transformation.* San Francisco, CA: Jossey-Bass.

Cantrell, M. (2008). The importance of debriefing in clinical simulations. *Clinical Simulation in Nursing, 4*(2), e19–e23.

Cronenwett, L., Sherwood, G., Barnsteiner, J., Disch, J., Johnson, J., Mitchell, P., et al. (2007). Quality and safety education for nurses. *Nursing Outlook, 55*(3), 122–131.

Henneman, E. H., & Cunningham, H. (2006). Using clinical simulation to teach patient safety in an acute/critical care nursing course. *Nurse Educator, 30*(4), 172–177.

Institute of Medicine. (2010). *The future of nursing: Leading change, advancing health.* Washington, DC: National Academies Press.

Lasater, K. (2007). Clinical judgment development: Using simulation to create an assess-ment rubric. *Journal of Nursing Education, 46*(11), 496–503.

Mariani, B., Cantrell, M. A., Meakim, C., Prieto, P., & Dreifuerst, K. T. (2013). Structured debriefing on students' clinical judgment abilities in simulation. *Clinical Simulation in Nursing Education, 9*(5), e147–e155.

Paparella, S., Mariani, B., Layton, K., & Carpenter, A. (2004). Patient safety simulation: Learning about safety never seemed so fun. *Journal for Nurses in Staff Development, 20*(6), 247–252.

Shinnick, M. A., Woo, M., Horwich, T. B., & Steadman, R. (2011). Debriefing: The most important component in simulation? *Clinical Simulation in Nursing, 7*(3), e105–e111.

Sears, K., Goldsworthy, S., & Goodman, W. M. (2010). The relationship between simulation in nursing education and medication safety. *Journal of Nursing Education, 49*(1), 52–55.

# 21

# Cultural Variations in End-of-Life Simulations

**Victoria R. Hammer,** EdD, MN, RN, CNE
**Susan M. Herm,** MSN, RN-BC
**Katherine A. Koepke,** MS, BSN, RN, CNHP

This innovative approach of students participating in a series of cultural end-of-life (EOL) simulations evolved during modifications in a second-semester baccalaureate clinical course titled Nursing Care of the Older Adult. The companion classroom course included EOL care as recommended by the End-of-Life Nursing Education Consortium (AACN, 2015), but there were no simulations relating to EOL. EOL care is an interaction that nurses may potentially encounter at some time in their career. It was noted in clinical that some nursing students had an opportunity to care for a patient at EOL and others did not. It was an emotional experience for those who did have this opportunity, and support from faculty was needed. Experiencing a patient death brings personal distress and feelings of inadequacy (Parry, 2011; Terry & Carroll, 2008). Providing a simulated EOL experience allows students to gain knowledge and skills in EOL care that could transfer into an authentic clinical setting (Radhakrishman, Roche, & Cunningham, 2007). This could decrease their initial distress of not knowing what to expect or what care to provide. A literature review found EOL simulations that included the "Silver Hour," which involved family, used faculty as standardized actors, used families and patients as actors, included interdisciplinary caregivers, and required students to act as nurses or observers (Crow, 2012; Pullen et al., 2012; Smith-Stoner, 2009; Twigg & Lynn, 2012).

The Silver Hour simulation was revised to cover one-half of the original time. The simulation included the time 30 minutes before and after death and involved the time from admission through the removal of the body from the site (Smith-Stoner, 2011). This time was decreased in the Silver Hour to include 15 minutes before and after death involving the time of imminent dying, the death, and the time immediately after death spent comforting the family and caring for the deceased body.

Our nursing students cared for individuals and families of several different cultures in various clinical settings in our community. Three of the cultures students encountered were Christian Caucasian, Native American, and Islam Somali. The racial demographics of this community from the 2010 census was recorded as 84.6 percent white, 7.8 percent black/African American, and 0.7 percent Native American. There has been an increasing Somali immigrant population in this community. Providing culturally competent care to individuals is expected in healthcare settings as a part of nursing care (Smith, 2013). This quality expectation extends to care at EOL and must be embedded into basic nursing education curriculum (Cronenwett, Sherwood, & Gelmon, 2009).

To prepare our students to provide culturally specific EOL care for those in our community, we created three different culturally appropriate EOL scenarios for a simulated clinical lab setting. Our goal was to complete three separate cultural EOL simulations in one clinical lab day. By doing so, the students would participate in or observe an EOL patient scenario in a simulated setting. In addition, they would compare and contrast how EOL care varied among three different cultures. Each nursing student has his or her own cultural set of beliefs regarding EOL care, but each must recognize that different cultures have their own approaches and rituals. To provide culturally competent EOL care, it is important to support the patient and family as they engage in their unique EOL practices, which may be different from the nurse's own cultural practices (Campinha-Bacote, 2011).

## DEVELOPMENT OF CULTURAL END-OF-LIFE SCENARIOS

Cultural EOL simulations were developed to include the three cultural groups of Christian Caucasian, Native American, and Islam Somali. Members from each culture and healthcare professionals were involved in the development of the scenarios. The faculty identified themselves as Christian Caucasian and sought recommendations from the Intervarsity Christian Fellowship chaplain and a hospice nurse. One faculty member met with the university's Native American Center director, who helped to create a Native American EOL scenario. One faculty member interacted with Somali community members and the university's Somali Student Association to gain their perspective on EOL in their culture. Faculty met with a Somali nurse, a former graduate of the nursing program, who helped to create the Islam Somali scenario. A hospice nurse was consulted for suggestions and to verify the accuracy of the scenes.

These simulations occurred on two consecutive days with groups of 20 to 40 students. The scenarios were scripted for a team of 4 students to provide culturally specific pre- and postmortem nursing care to the dying person and that person's family. Interdisciplinary healthcare team members were involved in this care. Non–role-players were assigned to observe and take notes. Each student was to participate in one scenario and observe two scenarios either by direct observation or via video-streaming of the scenario into a nearby classroom.

## STUDENTS, FACULTY, AND AUTHENTIC ACTORS

All actors were students, faculty, or volunteers from their cultural communities or interdisciplinary healthcare team members. Using the students as actors provided the opportunity to participate in and experience an EOL situation. Faculty as actors was helpful because they were aware of what would occur in the situations and could act the part (King & Ott, 2012). Using family members who have lived the experience provided authentic responses to situations that occurred in the simulation (Crow, 2012). Using the interdisciplinary healthcare team members allowed each to exhibit a role in EOL care, respond authentically in the scenarios, and demonstrate interdisciplinary collaboration to prepare the students for clinical practice (Pullen et al., 2012).

Students acted in the role of a nurse. Faculty acted as the reporting nurse or the voice of the patient/manikin. Faculty also controlled the high-tech manikin to respond as a dying patient might. In the Christian Caucasian scenario, the Intervarsity Christian Fellowship chaplain and hospice nurse who helped to develop the Christian Caucasian scenario participated as actors in their respective professional role. Three community women who had experienced the death of a close family member acted as daughters. Two of these women were from the Retired Senior Volunteer Program, and one was a retired nurse. In the Native American scenario, the Native American Center director who helped to develop the scenario and Native American students acted as family members. In the Islam Somali scenario, the Somali nurse who helped to develop this scenario contacted two Somali women familiar with Somali death rituals and an Imam. A Somali nurse acted as the granddaughter. The Imam provided spiritual support.

# PREPARING THE STUDENTS

The students engaged in 6 hours of classroom preparation, including discussions of loss, grief, bereavement, advance directives, and information regarding holistic pre- and postmortem care of the dying patient and the family (AACN, 2015). They completed their own advance directive and viewed the video *Dying Wish* (WordWise Productions, 2008). The students participated in a role-play about families facing decisions about an advance directive and care at the EOL. The students were given the objectives (Box 21.1) and assigned one cultural scenario. They searched for EOL information related to their assigned culture and shared this in class. On a discussion board, students posted their responses to the question, "Describe what you think would be most difficult for you as a nurse caring for an older adult near the end-of-life." In addition, there were discussions about EOL in clinical conferences.

---

## BOX 21.1

### Objectives: End-of-Life Simulation With Cultural Variations

1. Assess for physical signs at EOL such as dyspnea, bradycardia, mottling, cool touch, and dusky mouth color.
2. Exhibit caring behavior to the patient (manikin) and family (actors).
3. Adapt to cultural implications and rituals for EOL care (Christian Caucasian, Native American, Islam Somali)
4. Assess for advance directives and patient's wishes for before- and after-death care.
5. Provide comfort cares such as medications to relieve symptoms and control of pain and discomfort, skin care, turning, repositioning, and mouth care, including any other physical, psychological, social, and spiritual needs.
6. Participate in post-death care for patient (manikin).
7. Provide care of family (actors) and family needs (physical, psychological, social, and spiritual).
8. Reflect on EOL scenario simulation in debriefing sessions.

## PREPARING THE SCENE

In simulation, it is important to make the scene as real as possible (Jeffries, 2007; King & Ott, 2012; Merica, 2012; Smith-Stoner, 2009). To prepare the patient manikin to appear as a patient near death, the legs, feet, and hands were mottled with blue and red washable finger paint and dish soap. Briefs were moulaged with chocolate frosting covered with clear tape to simulate stool and yellow dish soap to simulate urine. The patient charts were modeled after hospice charts.

Christian Caucasian props included the Bible, cross, prayer shawl, flowers, and Christian music. Native American props included an amulet, a birch bark basket, sweet grass, and tobacco ties. The Native American actors wore traditional beadwork and vests. Props for the Islam Somali scenario included the Koran (Qur'an), prayer rug, hijab, a basin and pitcher for washing, and five sheets to wrap the deceased. The Somali women and Iman dressed in traditional attire.

## SIMULATION DAY

On the simulation day, the students and actors signed a consent form to be photographed/video-taped. The students wore their clinical scrubs. Students were gathered in their assigned groups according to culture and were randomly appointed a nurse role or an observer/note-taker role. The students decided how they were going to accomplish the nursing care as a team. They were introduced to the simulation room through a pre-briefing and received a change-of-shift report at the beginning of the simulation. The first time the simulations occurred, a low-tech manikin was used with the voice of a faculty member from behind a screen using a microphone to project the voice/breath of the patient. For the second and third simulations, a high-tech manikin in a simulation room was used, and the unfolding scenario was video-streamed into a nearby classroom to the nonparticipating students and a monitoring faculty member. This classroom was also set up as a debriefing room. Debriefing took place for 1 hour immediately after each simulation. The three cultural scenarios occurred consecutively on the same day.

## CULTURAL DIFFERENCES

It quickly became apparent there were definite cultural differences. Most students were Caucasian. The Christian scenario was chosen as the first scenario because it was more culturally familiar to the majority. When the Christian Caucasian patient was dying, the actor daughters shed tears, the chaplain read the Bible, and the hospice nurse altered medications and comforted the family. In the second scenario, the Native American family wanted tobacco ties on the bed and a smudging ceremony. They wanted the scene quiet so that the spirit of the dying person could go unhindered to the next world; and when this happened, the family joked, shared stories, and recalled fond memories of their loved one. The third scenario was the Islam Somali patient. Although the students had read about this culture's EOL rituals, they were awed at what transpired. The Islam Somali Imam read the Koran (Qur'an), and the Somali women carefully pressed the air and bodily contents out of the manikin, respectfully washed the deceased manikin three times, and wrapped it in five sheets for burial in 24 hours.

## DEBRIEFING AND CONTINUED LEARNING

Debriefing is a critical part of the simulation process, as it promotes the discovery of new knowledge and application to future situations (Jeffries, 2007). Faculty prepared themselves to lead the debriefing sessions by attending simulation conferences that included debriefing techniques and reading about how to lead debriefing sessions with sensitivity and empathy. The most effective debriefing occurs when the participants do most of the talking rather than the debriefing faculty (Jefferies). As suggested in the literature, the simulations were followed by a debriefing session that was double the time of each simulation (Smith-Stoner, 2009; Pullen et al., 2012; King & Ott, 2012; Lusk & Fater, 2013). Therefore, a 1-hour debriefing session was planned after each simulation. Those involved in the debriefing sessions included the faculty (who led the debriefing), the students, the participating healthcare professional, and the authentic actors. Including the authentic actors allowed further sharing of their lived experiences (Crow, 2012).

Debriefing sessions followed immediately after each simulation. All of the students, actors, and faculty sat in chairs placed in a large circle in the classroom. Coffee, juice, and treats were provided. In a nonthreatening and nonjudgmental manner, the debriefing faculty started with inquiring about the feelings of those present and what they had experienced. As the students shared their thoughts and feelings, emotions of past losses of those close to them surfaced. These feelings were accepted and supported. The group discussed what went well in the simulations, what could be improved, and how they could apply this in their future nursing care. The interdisciplinary healthcare actors shared their stories of caring for the dying and their families, what they had experienced, and the rationale for care. The cultural authentic actors participated by sharing their perspective(s), EOL rituals, and an explanation of cultural practices. A dynamic interchange of cultures transpired! Our students discovered how they could provide patient-centered EOL care within a cultural framework of EOL practices and rituals different from their own. This is the core of both patient centeredness and cultural competence (Campinha-Bacote, 2011).

## EVALUATION

A written evaluation followed immediately after the last debriefing session at the end of the day. Each student was given a form that listed the objectives, and each was asked to rate the objectives as met, partially met, or not met and to provide comments. On the back of this form, the students were asked to respond to these questions:

- "What were your feelings during each scenario?"
- "What went well?"
- "What would you change?"
- "What did you learn?"

Overall, most students stated that the objectives were met. Students expressed that the Christian Caucasian scenario was most familiar, brought feelings of sadness, and increased their knowledge of EOL care. They also stated that real emotions were evident and that the debriefing was beneficial. One student commented, "This simulation broadened my knowledge of EOL in all scenarios." Students stated that the Native American scenario helped them to gain information on Native American culture and to understand the minimal show of emotion and the journey to the next world. Some comments included:

- "I was not expecting the joking or not showing much emotion."
- "I learned that silence is ok."
- "Clear differences between cultures were presented."

Students thought that the Islam Somali scenario was interesting, respectful, showed family involvement, increased their knowledge of Somali culture, and was different from what they had experienced. They were unsure what to do. Comments included:

- "It felt awkward, but gave insights into cultural practice."
- "Their EOL care is so different than Christian Caucasian."

Overall, the students commented that they had expanded their learning about cultural differences at EOL. Some commented:

- "I learned more about the care of patients close to death from different cultures."
- "I feel more confident in assessing signs and symptoms that occur near death and how to communicate those findings with the family."
- "Debriefing was helpful to learn how to do the right thing in the future."
- "I learned how different each culture takes death, and how we as nurses need to be aware of those differences and be culturally sensitive."

## CONCLUSION

The cultural EOL simulations increased the students' awareness of differences in EOL care for patients and families in three cultures. Using members of the cultural communities and interdisciplinary professionals to develop and act in the scenarios made each scenario authentic and more real. The debriefing sessions provided the opportunity for students to acknowledge their feelings; expand their thinking, knowledge, and skills of culturally competent EOL care; and discuss future implications. We recommend using authentic cultural community members and interdisciplinary healthcare professionals to help develop and act in EOL simulations and participate in the debriefing sessions to enhance any EOL curriculum component in nursing education.

### References

American Association of Colleges of Nursing. (2015). *End-of-life nursing education consortium (ELNEC).* Retrieved June 20, 2015, from www.aacn.nche.edu/elnec

Campinha-Bacote, J. (2011). Delivering patient-centered care in midst of a cultural conflict: The role of cultural competence. *Online Journal of Issues in Nursing, 16*(2), 1.

Cronenwett, L., Sherwood, G., & Gelmon, S. B. (2009). Improving quality and safety education: The QSEN learning collaborative. *Nursing Outlook, 57*(6), 304–312.

Crow, K. M. (2012). Families and patients as actors in simulation: Adding unique perspectives to enhance nursing education. *Journal of Pediatric Nursing Education, 27*(6), 276–766.

Jeffries, P. R. (2007). *Simulation in nursing education: From conceptualization to evaluation.* New York, NY: National League for Nursing.

King, M. A., & Ott, J. (2012). Actors needed: Clinical faculty get the call. *Nurse Educator, 37*(3), 105–107.

Lusk, J. M., & Fater, K. (2013). Post-simulation debriefing to maximize clinical judgment development. *Nurse Educator, 38*(1), 16–19.

Merica, B. (2012). *Medical moulage: How to make your simulations come alive.* Philadelphia, PA: F. A. Davis.

Parry, M. (2011). Student nurses' experiences of their first death in clinical practice. *International Journal of Palliative Nursing, 17*(9), 448–453.

Pullen, R. L., McKelvy, K., Reyher, L., Thurman, J., Bencini, P., Taylor, T., et al. (2012). An end-of-life care interdisciplinary team clinical simulation model. *Nurse Educator, 37*(2), 75–79.

Radhakrishman, K., Roche, J. P., & Cunningham, H. M. (2007). Measuring clinical practice parameters with human patient simulation: A pilot study. *International Journal for Nursing Education Scholarship, 4*(1), 1–11.

Smith, L. S. (2013). Reaching for cultural competence. *Nursing, 43*(6), 30–38.

Smith-Stoner, M. (2009). Using high-fidelity simulation to educate nursing students about end-of-life care. *Nursing Education Perspectives, 30*(2), 115–120.

Smith-Stoner, M. (2011). Teaching patient-centered care during the silver hour. *Online Journal of Issues in Nursing, 16*(2), 1.

Terry, L. J., & Carroll, J. (2008). Dealing with death: First encounters for first-year nursing students. *British Journal of Nursing, 17*(12), 760–765.

Twigg, R. D., & Lynn, M. C. (2012). Teaching end-of-life care via a hybrid simulation approach. *Journal of Hospice & Palliative Nursing, 14*(5), 374–379.

WordWise Productions. (2008). *Dying wish.* Directed by Karen Van Vurren. Produced by Karen Van Vuuren and Francesca Nicosia. Boulder, CO: Author. Available from http://www.dyingwishmedia.com